Case Studies in
POLYSOMNOGRAPHY
INTERPRETATION

Case Studies in
POLYSOMNOGRAPHY
INTERPRETATION

Edited by

Robert C. Basner MD

Pulmonary, Critical Care, and Allergy Division,
Columbia University College of Physicians and Surgeons,
New York, USA

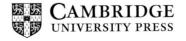

CAMBRIDGE UNIVERSITY PRESS
Cambridge, New York, Melbourne, Madrid, Cape Town,
Singapore, São Paulo, Delhi, Mexico City

Cambridge University Press

The Edinburgh Building, Cambridge CB2 8RU, UK

Published in the United States of America by
Cambridge University Press, New York

www.cambridge.org
Information on this title: www.cambridge.org/9781107015395

© Cambridge University Press 2012

First published 2012

Printed and Bound in the United Kingdom by the MPG Books Group

A catalogue record for this publication is available from the British Library

Library of Congress Cataloging-in-Publication Data

Case studies in polysomnography interpretation / [edited by] Robert C. Basner.
  p.   cm.
  ISBN 978-1-107-01539-5 (Hardback)
  1. Sleep disorders–Case studies.   2. Polysomnography–Case studies.
I. Basner, Robert C.
  RC547.C3738 2012
  616.8′498–dc23

2012020404

ISBN 978-1-107-01539-5 Hardback

Contents

Contributors

Robert C. Basner MD (cases 1–14)
Professor of Clinical Medicine in the Division of
Pulmonary, Allergy, and Critical Care Medicine, Columbia
University College of Physicians and Surgeons and
Director of the Cardiopulmonary Sleep and Ventilatory
Disorders Center, Columbia University Medical Center,
New York, USA

Carl Bazil MD PhD (cases 15–19)
Professor of Clinical Neurology and Director of the
Division of Epilepsy and Sleep, Columbia University
College of Physicians and Surgeons, New York, USA

Lee J. Brooks MD (cases 28 and 29)
Professor of Pediatrics, University of Pennsylvania and
Attending Physician at the Sleep Center of the Division of
Pulmonary Medicine, The Children's Hospital of
Philadelphia, Philadelphia, PA, USA

Sean M. Caples DO (cases 20–22)
Consultant, Center for Sleep Medicine, Division of
Pulmonary and Critical Care Medicine, Mayo Clinic,
Rochester, MN, USA

Kelly A. Carden MD (cases 23–27)
Center for Sleep, Sleep Medicine of Middle Tennessee, and
Saint Thomas Health, Nashville, TN, USA

Ronald D. Chervin MD MS (cases 47 and 48)
Professor of Neurology, the Michael S. Aldrich
Collegiate Professor of Sleep Medicine, and Director of the
University of Michigan Sleep Disorders Center,
Ann Arbor, MI, USA

Christopher Cielo DO (cases 28–31)
Fellow, Sleep Medicine and Pulmonology, Division of
Pulmonary Medicine, The Children's Hospital of
Philadelphia, Philadelphia, PA, USA

David G. Davila MD (case 32)
Baptist Health – Medical Center, Sleep Center Little Rock,
AR, USA

Katherine A. Dudley MD (cases 33–36)
Sleep Disorders Center, Beth Israel Deaconess Medical Center,
Harvard Medical School, Boston, MA, USA

Judy Fetterolf RPSGT REEGT (cases 102–104)
University of Michigan Health System Sleep Disorders Center,
Ann Arbor, MI, USA

W. Ward Flemons MD FRCPC (cases 92 and 93)
Professor of Medicine, University of Calgary, Alberta, Canada

Neil Freedman MD (cases 37–46)
Division of Pulmonary and Critical Care Medicine,
Department of Medicine, NorthShore University
HealthSystem, Evanston, IL, USA

Christian Guilleminault MD DBiol. (cases 105–107)
Stanford Sleep Medicine Division, Department of Psychiatry,
Stanford University School of Medicine, Redwood City,
CA, USA

Fauziya Hassan MD (cases 47 and 48)
Clinical Lecturer, University of Michigan, Ann Arbor,
MI, USA

Shelley Hershner MD (cases 49 and 50)
Assistant Professor of Neurology, University of Michigan,
Ann Arbor, MI, USA

David M. Hiestand MD PhD (cases 51–54)
Assistant Professor of Medicine and Director of the University
of Louisville Sleep Disorders Center, University of Louisville,
Louisville, KY, USA

Mithri Junna MD (cases 55 and 56)
Instructor in Neurology, Center for Sleep Medicine,
Departments of Neurology and Internal Medicine, Mayo
Clinic, Rochester, MN, USA

Kristen Kelly-Pieper MD (case 57)
Assistant Professor of Clinical Pediatrics, Division of Pediatric
Pulmonology, Columbia University College of Physicians and
Surgeons, New York, USA

Douglas Kirsch MD (cases 58 and 59)
Clinical Instructor, Harvard Medical School and Regional
Medical Director of the Sleep Health Centers,
Brighton, MA, USA

Brian B. Koo MD (cases 60 and 61)
Department of Neurology, Case Western Reserve University
School of Medicine, Cleveland, OH, USA

Carin Lamm MD (case 57)
Associate Clinical Professor of Pediatrics, Division of Pediatric
Pulmonology, Director, Pediatric Sleep Disorders Center,
Columbia University College of Physicians and Surgeons,
New York, USA

Raman Malhotra MD (cases 62–65)
Co-Director, SLU Care Sleep Disorders Center, Sleep
Medicine Fellowship Director, and Assistant Professor of
Neurology, Saint Louis University School of Medicine,
St. Louis, MO, USA

Meghna P. Mansukhani MBBS (case 66)
Center for Sleep Medicine, Mayo Clinic, Rochester, MN, USA

Carole L. Marcus MBBCh (cases 30 and 31)
Professor of Pediatrics, University of Pennsylvania and
Director of the Sleep Center, The Children's Hospital of
Philadelphia, Philadelphia, PA, USA

B. Marshall RPSGT (case 32)
Baptist Health – Medical Center, Sleep Center Little Rock,
AR, USA

Jean K. Matheson MD (cases 33, 67, and 68)
Associate Professor of Neurology, Division Head, Sleep
Medicine, Department of Neurology, Beth Israel Deaconess
Medical Center, Harvard Medical School, Boston, MA, USA

Timothy I. Morgenthaler MD (cases 55, 56, 66,
and 86)
Associate Professor of Medicine, Center for Sleep Medicine,
Mayo Clinic, Rochester, MN, USA

Gökhan M. Mutlu MD (cases 69–77)
Associate Professor of Medicine, Northwestern University
Feinberg School of Medicine, Chicago, IL, USA

Irina Ok MD (cases 78–84)
City University of New York (CUNY), New York, USA

Vidya Pai MD (case 85)
Fellow in Sleep Medicine, Center for Pediatric Sleep
Disorders, Children's Hospital, Boston, MA, USA

Winnie C. Pao MD (case 86)
Center for Sleep Medicine, Mayo Clinic, Rochester, MN, USA

Sairam Parthasarathy MD (cases 87–91)
Associate Professor of Medicine, Director, Center for Sleep
Disorders, University of Arizona, Tucson, AZ, USA

Shalini Paruthi MD (cases 62–65)
Clinical Assistant Professor of Pediatrics and Internal
Medicine, Saint Louis University School of Medicine and
Director of the Pediatric Sleep and Research Center,
St. Louis, MO, USA

Nimesh Patel DO (cases 87–91)
Fellow in Pulmonary and Critical Care Medicine, University
of Arizona, Tucson, AZ, USA

Sachin R. Pendharkar MD MSc FRCPC (cases 92
and 93)
Assistant Professor of Medicine, University of Calgary,
Calgary, Canada

Ravi K. Persaud MPH (cases 1–14)
Chief Technologist, Cardiopulmonary Sleep and Ventilatory
Disorders Center, Columbia University Medical Center,
New York, USA

Bharati Prasad MD (case 94)
Assistant Professor of Medicine, University of Illinois at
Chicago, Chicago, IL, USA

Stuart F. Quan MD (cases 95 and 96)
Gerald E. McGinnis Professor of Sleep Medicine, Division of
Sleep Medicine, Harvard Medical School, Boston, MA, USA

Satish C. Rao MD MS (case 51)
Medical Director of Neurosciences Services, Floyd Memorial
Hospital, New Albany, IN, USA

Patti Reed RPSGT (case 32)
Baptist Health – Medical Center, Sleep Center Little Rock,
AR, USA

Alcibiades Rodriguez MD FAASM (cases 78–84)
Medical Director, New York Sleep Institute, Divisional
Director of Sleep Disorders, Department of Neurology,
Assistant Professor of Neurology, NYU School of Medicine,
New York, USA

Dennis Rosen MD (cases 85, 97, and 98)
Assistant Professor of Pediatrics, Harvard Medical
School and Associate Medical Director of the Center for
Pediatric Sleep Disorders, Children's Hospital, Boston,
MA, USA

Vijay Seelall MD (cases 99 and 100)
Director of Sleep Medicine, Beth Israel Medical Center,
Assistant Professor, Albert Einstein College of Medicine,
New York, NY, USA

Anita Valanju Shelgikar MD (case 101)
Clinical Instructor of Neurology, Program Director, and
Sleep Medicine Fellow, University of Michigan, Ann Arbor,
MI, USA

Jeffrey J. Stanley MD (cases 102–104)
Assistant Professor, University of Michigan Health System,
Ann Arbor, MI, USA

Kingman Strohl MD (cases 60, 61, and 111)
Department of Neurology, Case Western Reserve University
School of Medicine, Cleveland, OH, USA

Shannon S. Sullivan MD (cases 105–107)
Stanford Sleep Medicine Division, Department of Psychiatry, Stanford University School of Medicine, Redwood City, CA, USA

Kevin A. Thomas RPSGT (cases 52–54)
Technical Director, Pediatric Sleep Laboratory, University of Louisville, Louisville, KY, USA

Robert Thomas MD MMSc (cases 34–36)
Assistant Professor of Medicine, Harvard Medical School, Beth Israel Deaconess Medical Center, Boston, MA, USA

John R. Wheatley MB BS(Hons) PhD FRACP (cases 108–110)
Professor of Medicine, University of Sydney and Director of Respiratory and Sleep Medicine, Westmead Hospital, Sydney, Australia

Lisa Wolfe MD (cases 69–77)
Division of Pulmonary and Critical Care Medicine, Northwestern University Feinberg School of Medicine, Chicago, IL, USA

Peter J.-C. Wu MB BS (Hons) BSc(Med) FRACP (cases 108–110)
Staff Specialist, Department of Respiratory and Sleep Medicine, Westmead Hospital, Sydney, Australia

Motoo Yamauchi MD (case 111)
Visiting Fellow, UH Case Medical Center, Cleveland, OH, USA

Preface

This volume began as a series of workshops in polysomnogram interpretation and is intended to afford the reader a unique opportunity to match her/his own expertise and interest in interpreting polysomnograms with national and international expert polysomnographers. The authors, experts in adult and pediatric sleep medicine, offer examples of important polysomnograms and clinical cases directly from their own sleep laboratories: not idealized or touched up, these are the "real life" tracings as they were recorded.

The authors have provided detailed descriptions of their interpretative thought processes as well as relevant references, such that the reader is able to, in a sense, sit with these experts as they work through their own interpretations. By design, many of the incorrect choices the reader is offered look appealing and plausible, and often the precise answer turns on a master point of view rather than any hard and fast "rule." The authors do not, however, claim that theirs is the only possible interpretation of the tracings and data which appear here: polysomnogram interpretation is an art as well as a science. It is also stressed that the terms "correct" and "incorrect," which accompany each case in this volume, refer to a specific expert author's interpretation of the polysomnogram displayed in the clinical setting in which it was created. The reader may well have an explanation that differs from the author's as presented here, and to the extent that it is a rational and justified interpretation, this volume will have done its job: encouraging expert and refined consideration and analysis of vital aspects of polysomnography.

Because we have stressed the reader's ability to form her/his own interpretation of the polysomnogram tracing in the context of the case, we have not provided a traditional format of topics and chapters. Rather, we have arranged cases in alphabetical order of the first author and have provided a table of contents with a short title for each case history. In this way, we expect that as the reader works through a specific authors' cases and polysomnogram examples (arranged in alphabetical order), she/he will come to the cases and polysomnogram examples with the challenge of the interpretation intact, without a prior knowledge regarding whether the case primarily depicts a respiratory, cardiac, neurologic, circadian, or parasomnia disorder, although there will be certain natural clustering of cases from some authors. The reader will also be able to consult the index to pursue a specific type of abnormality if she/he prefers that style of working through these cases.

The reader is encouraged to form her/his own answer prior to checking the authors' interpretation of correct and incorrect answers, which appear in the second part of the book (pp. 137–206).

The interpretations and clinical suggestions herein are strictly the opinion of the authors; such interpretations may not necessarily apply to a specific patient of the reader's, and the intent here is expressly not treatment but polysomnogram interpretation, although it is important that the context of the interpretation be fully understood and accounted for.

Further, this volume is not specifically designed as a "board review" of sleep medicine. Nevertheless, it is expected that the reader who is able to work through the correct and incorrect interpretations of the polysomnograms displayed in these cases in a thorough and reasoned fashion will have gone far in attaining important and relevant expertise in all of these aspects of sleep medicine, and should be able to bring enhanced and indeed commanding skills to any examination situation, as well as to the interpretation of polysomnograms in her/his own practice.

I thank each of the authors, who contributed their expertise, time, and devotion to teaching and polysomnographic reasoning to create this volume, and the publishers, particularly Jane Seakins and Nicholas Dunton, whose insight, collaboration, and hard work was invaluable in bringing this text to the form in front of you.

We welcome your comments and suggestions regarding this format and the topics and interpretations herein. Good interpretation, and good health to your patients.

Robert C. Basner, MD
Columbia University College of Physicians and Surgeons
New York City, USA

FURTHER READING

American Academy of Sleep Medicine. *International Classification of Sleep Disorders, Diagnostic and Coding Manual*, 2nd edn. Westchester, IL: American Academy of Sleep Medicine, 2005.

Iber C, Ancoli-Israel S, Chesson A for the American Academy of Sleep Medicine. *The AASM Manual for the Scoring of Sleep and Associated Events: Rules, Terminology, and Technical Specifications*. Westchester, IL: American Academy of Sleep Medicine, 2007.

Abbreviations

A1	left mastoid (ear) referential EEG	F4 (F4-M, F4-A)	right frontal referential EEG
A2	right mastoid (ear) referential EEG	FLOW	airflow derived from pressure signal
Abd/Abdo (ABD, ABDO, ABDOMEN, ABDM, Abdm8)	abdominal respiratory inductance plethysmography	Fz-Cz	midline frontal, central EEG
		HR	heart rate
AHI	apnea hypopnea index	ICSD	International Classification of Sleep Disorders
AASM	American Academy of Sleep Medicine	IPAP	inspiratory positive airway pressure
AV	atrioventricular	L Leg (LLEG, Lleg)	left pretibial EMG
BMI	body mass index	LAT	left anterior tibialis EMG
C2 (C2-M, C2-A)	right central referential EEG	LEOG	left eye referential EOG
C3 (C3-M, C3-A)	left central referential EEG	LOC	left eye referential EOG
C4 (C4-M, C4-A)	right central referential EEG	MRI	magnetic resonance imaging
CFLOW	airflow derived from pressure signal	MSLT	multiple sleep latency test
		MWT	maintenance of wakefulness test
CHEST	thoracic respiratory inductance plethysmography	N/O	oronasal thermistor
Chest/Abd	thoracic and abdominal respiratory inductance plethysmography	NAF	nasal pressure transducer
		Nasal Press (NPress, Nasal P)	nasal pressure transducer
		NPRE	nasal pressure transducer
Chin, CHN	submental EMG	NREM	non-rapid eye movement
CO2 wave	end-tidal partial pressure CO_2 ($ETco_2$)	O1 (O1-M, O1-A)	left occipital referential EEG
		O2 (O2-M, O2-A)	right occipital referential EEG
COPD	chronic obstructive pulmonary disease	OSA	obstructive sleep apnea
CPAP	continuous positive airway pressure	OSAT	O_2 saturation by oximetry (Spo_2)
CPRESS	positive airway pressure signal (positive deflection upwards)	$Paco_2$	partial pressure of CO_2 arterial
		Pao_2	partial pressure of O_2 arterial
		PAP flow	airflow derived from pressure signal
Cz-Oz	midline central, occipital EEG	PAP	positive airway pressure
E1 (E1-M)	left referential EOG	PFlow (PFLOW, PFLO)	nasal air pressure transducer
E2 (E2-M)	right referential EOG	PLM	periodic limb movement
ECG/EKG	electrocardiogram	PSG	polysomnography/ polysomnogram
ECGL-ECGR	precordial ECG		
EEG	electroencephalography/ electroencephalogram	PTAF	nasal pressure transducer
		Pulse	pulse rate from pulse oximetry
EMG Tib	right and left leg EMG	R Leg (RLEG, Rleg)	right pretibial EMG
EMG	electromyography/ electromyogram	RAT	right anterior tibialis EMG
		RBD	REM sleep behavior disorder
EOG	electro-oculography/electro-oculogram	REM	rapid eye movement
		RERA	respiratory effort-related arousal
EPAP	expiratory positive airway pressure	REOG	right eye referential EOG
		ROC	right eye referential EOG
$ETco_2$	end-tidal partial pressure CO_2	RLS	restless leg syndrome
F3 (F3-M, F3-A)	left frontal referential EEG		

Snore (SNORE, Snore5, PSnore, SNOR)	snoring channel	TCco$_2$	transcutaneous CO$_2$
Sono	snoring channel	Therm (THERM, Therm6)	airflow via oronasal thermistor
SOREM	sleep-onset REM sleep	Tho (THO, THOR, Thorax7)	thoracic respiratory inductance plethysmography
Spo$_2$ (Sao$_2$)	O$_2$ saturation by oximetry		
SSRI	selective serotonin reuptake inhibitor		
Sum (sum, SUM)	summation of abdominal and thoracic respiratory inductance plethysmography		

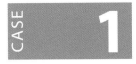

CASE 1

A 74-year-old man with severe ischemic cardiomyopathy and atrial fibrillation

Robert C. Basner, with technical assistance from Ravi K. Persaud

The following 3 minute polysomnogram (PSG) tracing was recorded in a 74-year-old man with severe ischemic cardiomyopathy and atrial fibrillation. His awake arterial blood gases breathing room air at sea level are PaO_2 of 70 mmHg and $PaCO_2$ of 38 mmHg. The tracing represents the patient breathing room air.

What is the best interpretation of the respiratory status of this patient displayed on this tracing?
A. Cheyne–Stokes breathing
B. Hypoventilation
C. Hypopneas
D. Respiratory effort-related arousals (RERAs)
E. Normal rapid eye movement (REM)-related breathing.

Answer on page 138.

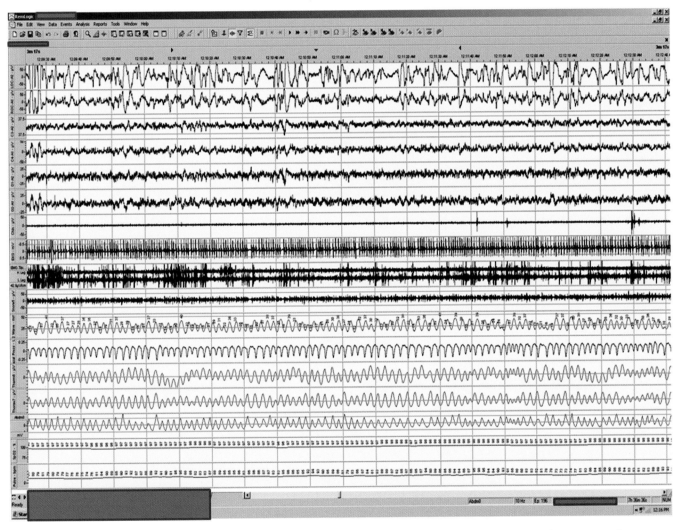

A1, left mastoid (ear) referential electroencephalography (EEG); A2, right mastoid (ear) referential EEG; Abdm8, abdominal respiratory inductance plethysmography; ECG, electrocardiogram (precordial right-sided); C3, left central referential EEG; C4, right central referential EEG; Chin, submental electromyogram (EMG); EMG Tib, right and left leg EMG; LOC, left eye referential electro-oculogram (EOG); Nasal Press, nasal pressure transducer; O1, left occipital referential EEG; O2, right occipital referential EEG; Pulse, pulse rate from pulse oximeter; ROC, right eye referential EOG; Spo2, O_2 saturation by oximetry (from ear pulse oximetry); Therm6, oronasal thermistor; Thorax7, thoracic respiratory inductance plethysmography; 2 Wave, end-tidal PCO_2 ($ETCO_2$). Highest $ETCO_2$ value displayed (11th channel from top) is 41 mmHg; Nadir Spo_2 displayed (2nd channel from bottom) is 96%.

Case Studies in Polysomnography Interpretation, ed. Robert C. Basner. Published by Cambridge University Press. © Cambridge University Press 2012.

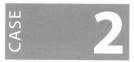

CASE 2

A 65-year-old man with amyotrophic lateral sclerosis

Robert C. Basner, with technical assistance from Ravi K. Persaud

The 60 second PSG epoch displayed below was recorded in a 65-year-old man with amyotrophic lateral sclerosis. The patient is supine and being ventilated with bilevel positive airway pressure (PAP) at 10 cmH$_2$O inspiratory PAP (IPAP) and 4 cmH$_2$O expiratory PAP (EPAP) using a hybrid (mouthpiece plus nasal prongs) interface.

Which of the following is the most likely maneuver performed by the technician at the notation "EVENT" (2:24:05 a.m.)?

A. The setting was changed from ST (spontaneous/timed) mode with back-up rate of 20/minute to S (spontaneous mode) without a back-up rate

B. Supplementary O$_2$ was added in-line to an adapter just below the interface at 4 L/min flow rate

C. The thoracic and abdominal respiratory inductance plethysmography belts were tightened to allow for a better signal

D. The trigger sensitivity was changed from high to low in ST mode, with a continued back-up rate of 12/minute

E. The bilevel PAP was changed to continuous PAP (CPAP) of 4 cmH$_2$O.

Answer on page 138.

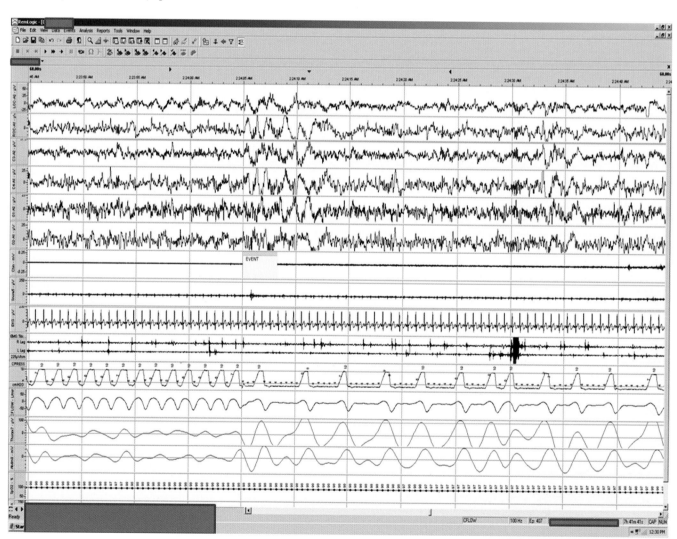

C2, right central referential EEG; CFLOW, airflow derived from pressure signal; CPRESS, PAP signal, positive deflection upwards (5th channel from bottom).

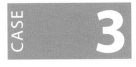

An 80-year-old man with severe heart failure and witnessed apnea awake and during sleep

Robert C. Basner, with technical assistance from Ravi K. Persaud

The following 60 second PSG tracing was recorded in an 80-year-old man with severe heart failure and witnessed apneas awake and during sleep.

How is the respiratory event depicted in the middle of the epoch best interpreted?
A. Obstructive apnea during CPAP titration
B. Central apnea during servo bilevel PAP ventilation
C. Hypopnea during spontaneous breathing
D. Hypopnea during fixed bilevel PAP ventilation
E. None of the above.

Answer on page 139.

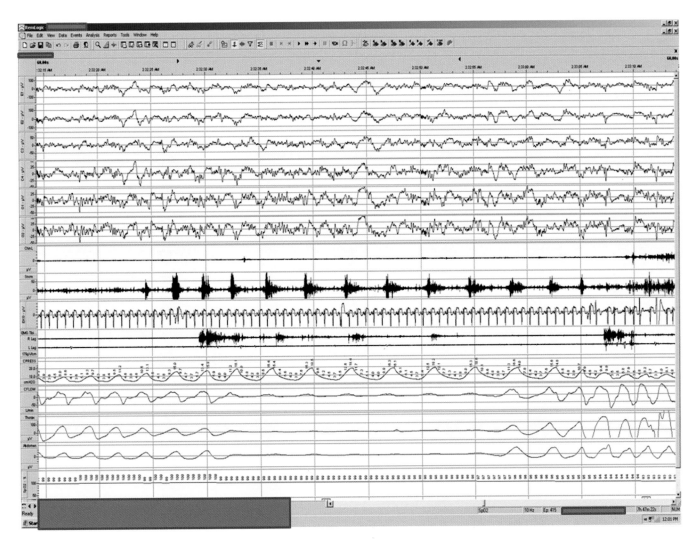

Abdomen, abdominal respiratory inductance plethysmography; E1, E2, left and right referential EOG; Thorax, thoracic respiratory inductance plethysmography; Spo₂ by ear pulse oximetry. PAP is 5th channel up from bottom.

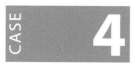

CASE 4

A 33-year-old man with a history of interstitial pulmonary fibrosis and obesity

Robert C. Basner, with technical assistance from Ravi K. Persaud

The following 60 second epoch is from a PSG recorded in a 33-year-old man with a history of interstitial pulmonary fibrosis and obesity, who was studied to assess for a sleep-related breathing disorder and the need for PAP therapy. The patient is receiving supplemental O_2 at 4 L/min via nasal cannulae.

What is the best interpretation of the right-sided precordial ECG (8th channel from the top) displayed here?
A. Sinus rhythm with right bundle branch block
B. Ventricular tachycardia
C. Atrial flutter with 2:1 conduction
D. Hyperkalemia effect
E. Artifact.

Answer on page 140.

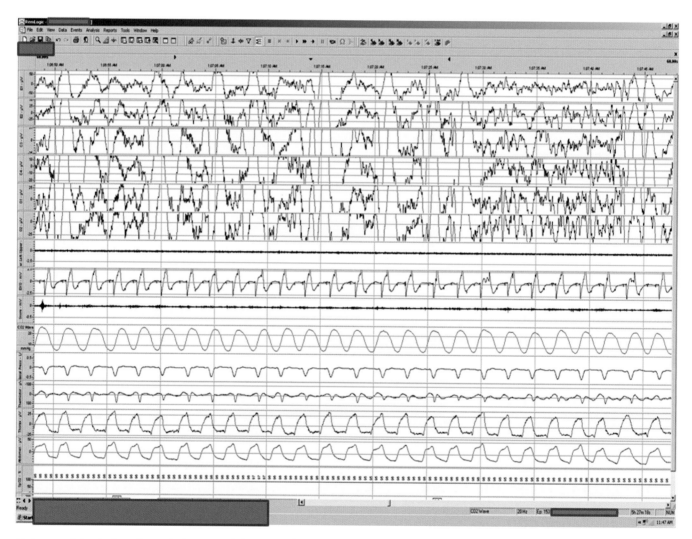

Abdomen, abdominal respiratory inductance plethysmography; Er, Left-upper, submental EMG; Thorax, thoracic respiratory inductance plethysmography; Spo2 by ear pulse oximetry. ECG tracing is 8th channel from the top.

A 52-year-old man being treated for sleep-related hypoventilation

Robert C. Basner, with technical assistance from Ravi K. Persaud

A 30 second PSG epoch is shown that was recorded in a 52-year-old man being treated for sleep-related hypoventilation with bilevel nasal PAP of 14 cmH$_2$O IPAP and 6 cmH$_2$O EPAP.

Which of the following best describes the ECG displayed?
A. Ashman phenomenon
B. Sinus arrhythmia
C. Junctional rhythm
D. Sinus rhythm with first-degree atrioventricular (AV) block
E. Sinus rhythm with frequent premature supraventricular beats.

Answer on page 141.

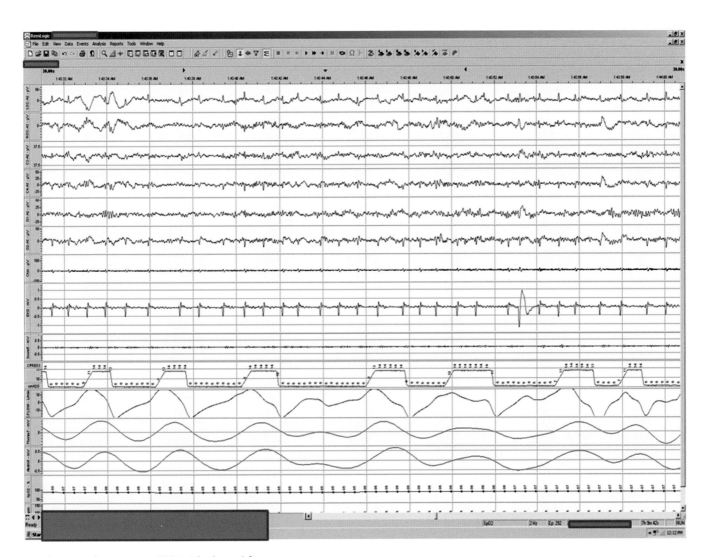

Spo$_2$ by ear pulse oximetry; ECG is 8th channel from top.

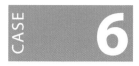

An 81-year-old obese woman with a history of snoring

Robert C. Basner, with technical assistance from Ravi K. Persaud

Displayed below is a 60 second PSG epoch of supine sleep recorded in an 81-year-old woman with a body mass index (BMI) of 31 and a history of snoring, who is being assessed for a sleep-related breathing disorder. She is breathing room air. Her awake arterial blood gas when breathing room air prior to the study was Pao_2 of 77 mmHg and $Paco_2$ of 40 mmHg.

What is the best interpretation of the respiratory status as depicted here as consistent with the AASM Manual?
A. Snoring alone
B. Hypoventilation
C. Respiratory effort-related arousals
D. REM-related hypoxemia
E. Complex sleep apnea.

Answer on page 141.

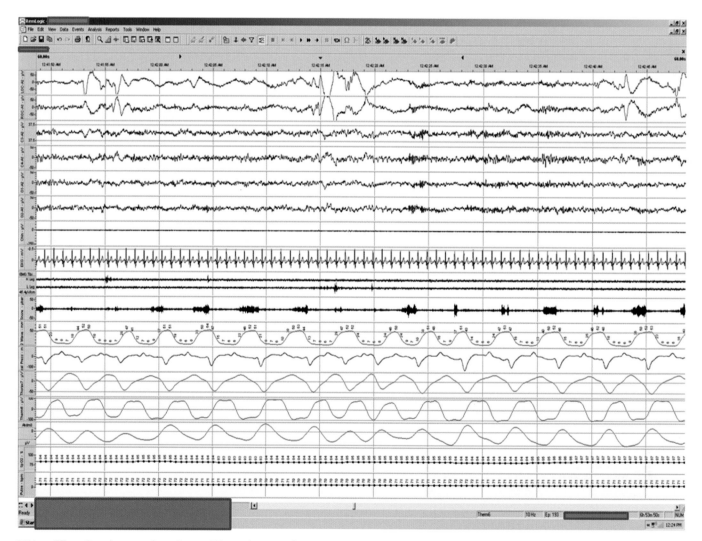

2 Wave, $ETco_2$; Spo_2 by ear pulse oximetry. $ETco_2$ values vary from 47 to 54 mmHg, and are generally 75 mmHg as displayed. Spo_2 values are in the 93–94% range.

Case Studies in Polysomnography Interpretation, ed. Robert C. Basner. Published by Cambridge University Press. © Cambridge University Press 2012.

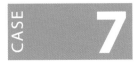

A 33-year-old obese man with idiopathic pulmonary fibrosis and snoring

CASE 7

Robert C. Basner, with technical assistance from Ravi K. Persaud

The following 60 second epoch of non-REM (NREM) sleep is from a PSG recording in a 33-year-old man with a BMI of 35, snoring, and idiopathic pulmonary fibrosis awaiting lung transplant.

What is the best PSG interpretation of the cause of the hypoxemia depicted on this tracing?
A. Hypoventilation
B. Obstructive sleep apnea (OSA)
C. Snoring alone
D. Artifact
E. Complex sleep apnea.

Answer on page 142.

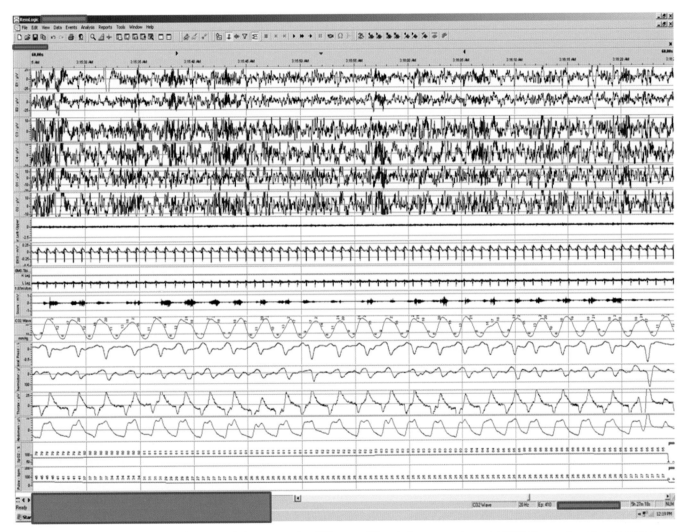

Abdomen, abdominal respiratory inductance plethysmography; CO2 wave, ETco$_2$; Left-upper, submental EMG; Thorax, thoracic respiratory inductance plethysmography; Spo$_2$ by ear pulse oximetry. Spo$_2$ values are in the high 70 to mid 80% range (2nd channel from bottom). ETco$_2$ (7th channel from bottom) is < 30 mmHg throughout tracing. Pulse is displayed as the bottommost channel and shows values of ⩽ 45 bpm throughout the tracing.

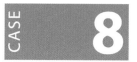
A 57-year-old woman with moderate obstructive sleep apnea

Robert C. Basner, with technical assistance from Ravi K. Persaud

The following is a 30 second epoch from a nocturnal PSG performed in a 57-year-old woman with moderate OSA undergoing titration with CPAP.

Which one of the following parameters present in this tracing is both necessary and sufficient to score this epoch as stage R (REM) sleep?

A. Low-amplitude, mixed frequency EEG
B. REMs
C. Low chin EMG tone
D. Sawtooth waves
E. Irregular shallow airflow and breathing efforts
F. None of the above.

Answer on page 142.

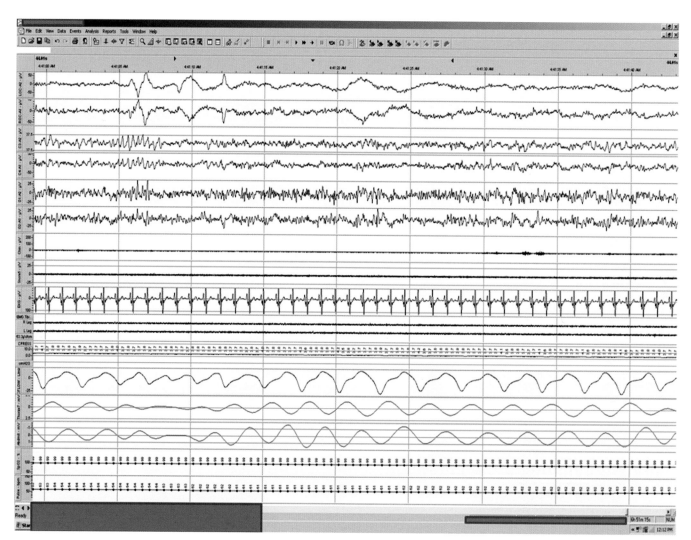

R leg, L leg, pretibial EMG, right and left respectively; Spo₂ by ear pulse oximetry.

Case Studies in Polysomnography Interpretation, ed. Robert C. Basner. Published by Cambridge University Press. © Cambridge University Press 2012.

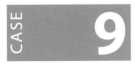
A 57-year-old woman with potential obstructive sleep apnea

Robert C. Basner, with technical assistance from Ravi K. Persaud

The following is a 60 second PSG tracing from a 57-year-old woman being studied to assess for OSA. Her awake baseline $ETco_2$ was 38 mmHg. The tracing occurs with the patient supine in REM sleep.

What is the best interpretation of the respiratory event which occurs between 1:38:40 a.m. and 1:39:00 a.m.?
A. Obstructive apnea only
B. Hypopnea only
C. Hypoventilation only
D. Respiratory effort-related arousal only
E. Mixed apnea only
F. Any of A, B or C can be scored by current scoring rules.

Answer on page 143.

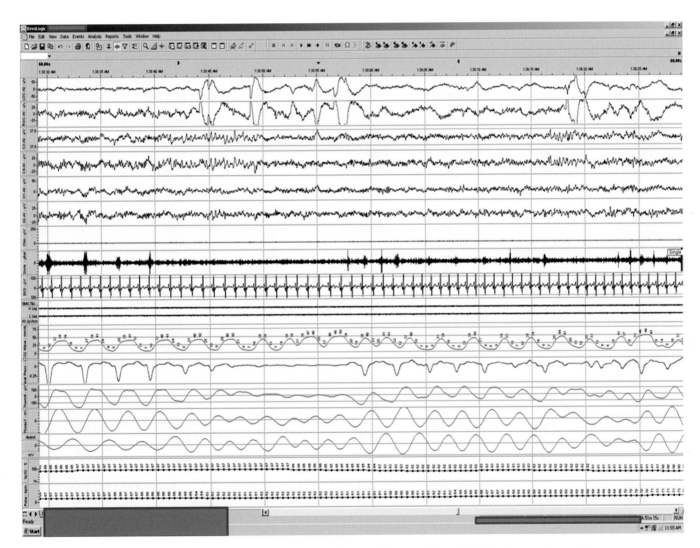

Spo_2 from ear pulse oximetry (2nd channel from bottom). Spo_2 nadir is 92% (decreased from 97%) for the event in question.

Case Studies in Polysomnography Interpretation, ed. Robert C. Basner. Published by Cambridge University Press. © Cambridge University Press 2012.

An 80-year-old man with heart failure and previously documented Cheyne–Stokes breathing

Robert C. Basner, with technical assistance from Ravi K. Persaud

The following 5 minute PSG tracing was recorded during NREM sleep with the application of servo PAP ventilation in an 80-year-old man with heart failure and previously documented Cheyne–Stokes breathing. The patient is supine using a hybrid (oral mask with nasal prongs) interface. The technician notes a large air leak at the time of this tracing. The back-up rate for the ventilation is 15 breaths/min.

What is the best interpretation of the respiratory status of this patient based on the displayed tracing?

A. Cheyne–Stokes breathing
B. Patient–ventilator asynchrony
C. Mixed apneas
D. Expected response to servo ventilation in NREM sleep
E. None of the above.

Answer on page 144.

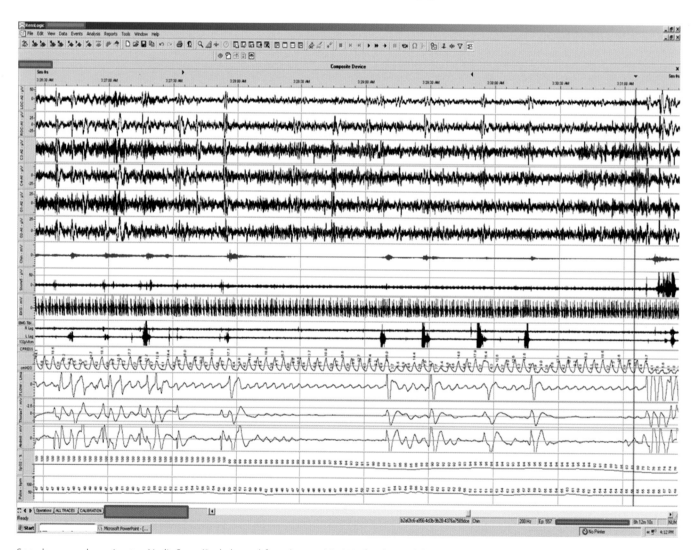

Spo_2 by ear pulse oximetry. Nadir Spo_2 (2nd channel from bottom) is 85% for the middle respiratory event, and 74% for the last respiratory event shown.

Case Studies in Polysomnography Interpretation, ed. Robert C. Basner. Published by Cambridge University Press. © Cambridge University Press 2012.

A 46-year-old obese man with loud snoring, witnessed apnea, and daytime sleepiness

Robert C. Basner, with technical assistance from Ravi K. Persaud

The following two precordial ECG tracings were recorded during a single night of PSG in an obese 46-year-old man with loud snoring, witnessed apneas, and daytime sleepiness. Figure 1A is a 60 minute tracing in NREM sleep beginning at approximately 10:52 p.m.; Figure 1B is a 30 minute tracing in NREM sleep beginning approximately 3 a.m.

What is the best interpretation of the event that took place between the two tracings?

A. Application of an external pacemaker for sick sinus syndrome
B. Spontaneous resolution of Wolff–Parkinson–White syndrome associated tachyarrhythmia
C. Resumption of paced rhythm via permanent pacemaker after pacemaker failure failure
D. Application of CPAP.

Answer on page 144.

A

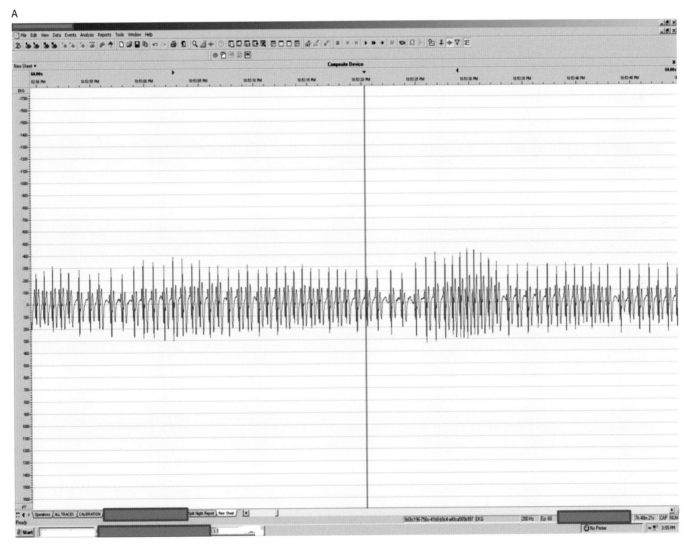

Fig. 1.

B

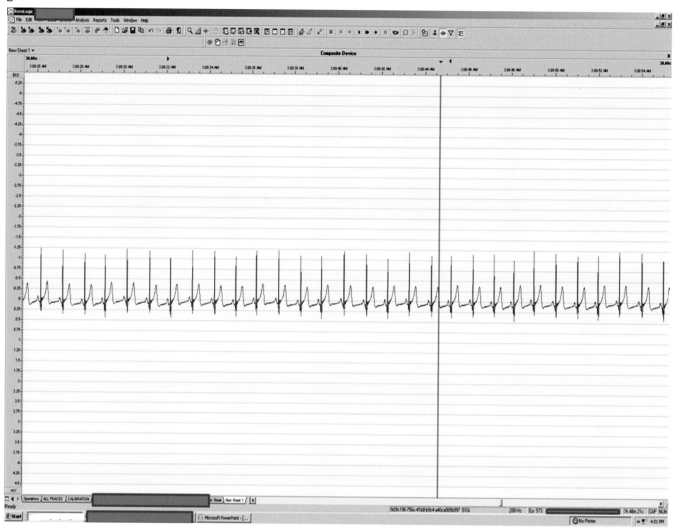

Fig. 1 (cont.)

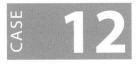

A 60-year-old woman with severe obstructive sleep apnea

Robert C. Basner, with technical assistance from Ravi K. Persaud

The following approximately 24 second PSG tracing of REM (stage R) sleep was recorded in a 60-year-old woman with severe OSA.

1. **What is the best interpretation of the respiratory findings seen on this tracing?**
A. Complex apnea during CPAP use
B. Obstructive apnea during bilevel PAP use
C. Mixed apnea during bilevel PAP use
D. Hypoventilation during CPAP use
E. Central apnea during spontaneous breathing.

2. **What is the best interpretation of the ECG in the above PSG tracing?**
A. Sinus rhythm with a period of second-degree AV block
B. Sinus rhythm with first-degree AV block
C. Sinus rhythm with a period of third-degree AV block
D. Atrial fibrillation during the apnea; atrial flutter following the apnea.

Answer on page 146.

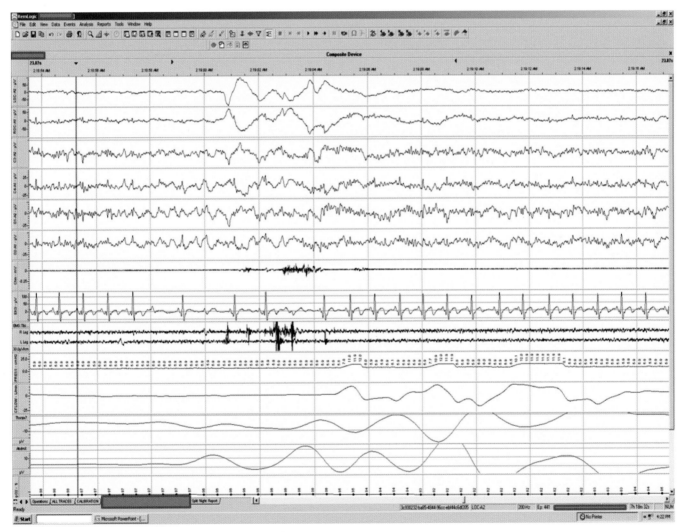

Spo₂ from ear pulse oximetry (bottommost channel). Nadir Spo₂ is 92%.

Case Studies in Polysomnography Interpretation, ed. Robert C. Basner. Published by Cambridge University Press. © Cambridge University Press 2012.

A 52-year-old man with valvular cardiomyopathy

Robert C. Basner, with technical assistance from Ravi K. Persaud

The following 60 second PSG tracing of NREM sleep was recorded in a 52-year-old man with valvular cardiomyopathy (left ventricular ejection fraction, 20%). The patient's awake $Paco_2$ supine is 34 mmHg.

Based upon the AASM Manual, what is the best interpretation of the respiratory event on this tracing?

A. Central apnea
B. Mixed apnea
C. Cheyne–Stokes breathing
D. Hypoventilation
E. There is not enough information to accurately score this event.

Answer on page 147.

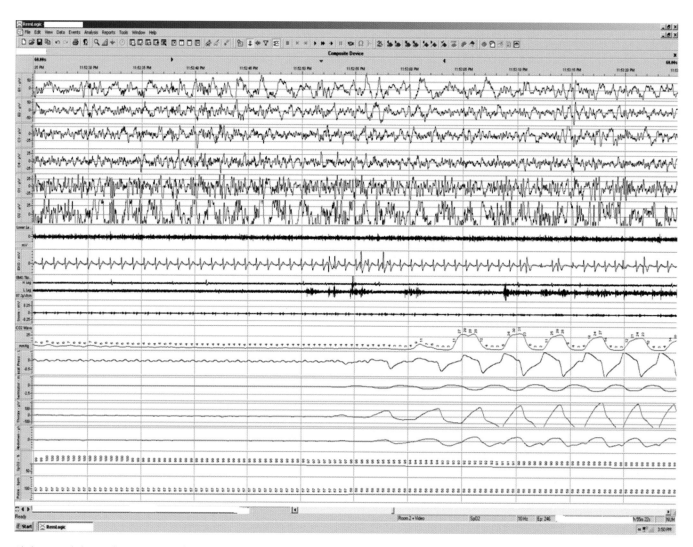

Abdomen, abdominal respiratory inductance plethysmography; Lower left upper, submental EMG; Thorax, thoracic respiratory inductance plethysmography; Spo_2 from ear pulse oximetry (2nd channel from bottom). $ETco_2$ is 7th channel from bottom (maximum depicted here is 39 mmHg).

Case Studies in Polysomnography Interpretation, ed. Robert C. Basner. Published by Cambridge University Press. © Cambridge University Press 2012.

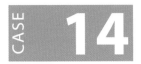

CASE 14

An otherwise healthy 40-year-old man with potential obstructive sleep apnea

Robert C. Basner, with technical assistance from Ravi K. Persaud

The following is a 30 second representative PSG tracing in NREM sleep (stage N3) in an otherwise healthy 40-year-old man being studied to assess for OSA.

What is the most accurate interpretation of the precordial ECG seen on this tracing?

A. Respiratory sinus arrhythmia
B. Electrical alternans
C. Pulsus alternans
D. Movement artifact
E. Total alternans.

Answer on page 148.

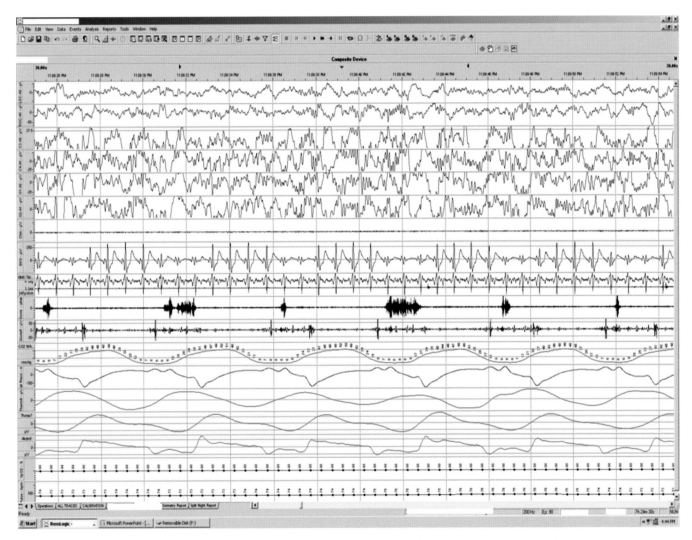

Abdm, abdominal respiratory inductance plethysmography; CO2 wa, ETco$_2$ (mmHg); Thorax, thoracic respiratory inductance plethysmography; Spo$_2$ from ear pulse oximetry. ECG is the 8th channel from the top of the trace. The one immediately below is the tibialis EMG (left upper, right lower).

A 32-year-old man with observed severe snoring and leg shaking during sleep

Carl Bazil

The following 30 second PSG tracing was recorded in a 32-year-old man with observed severe snoring, and leg shaking during sleep. Medications at the time of the recording included phenytoin.

What is the interpretation of the event indicated at the arrow, seen in the EEG and EOG channels?

A. Electrographic arousal
B. Movement artifact
C. Generalized spike-wave discharge
D. Snoring artifact
E. Posterior dominant rhythm.

Answer on page 148.

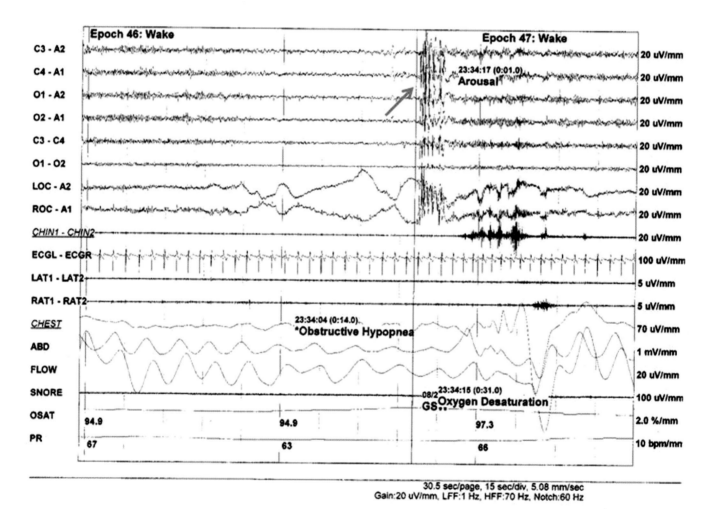

CHEST, thoracic respiratory inductance plethysmography; ECGL-ECGR, precordial ECG; LAT, left anterior tibialis EMG; OSAT, Spo₂ (by ear pulse oximetry); RAT, right anterior tibialis EMG.

Case Studies in Polysomnography Interpretation, ed. Robert C. Basner. Published by Cambridge University Press. © Cambridge University Press 2012.

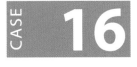

CASE 16 — A 20-year-old woman with extreme sleepiness who reports hypnic hallucinations, sleep paralysis, and sudden loss of muscle tone when startled

Carl Bazil

A 20-year-old woman was referred for extreme sleepiness that began over the previous month. She frequently falls asleep in unusual places, including on the toilet. Additionally, she reports hypnic hallucinations, sleep paralysis, and sudden loss of muscle tone when startled. The hypnogram from her overnight PSG is shown below. No significant respiratory events or periodic limb movements (PLMs) were seen on the overnight study.

Based on the history and interpretation of the hypnogram, which of the following is least consistent with a diagnosis of narcolepsy here?
A. Extreme sleepiness
B. Relatively sudden onset at age 20
C. Loss of muscle tone with startle
D. The sleep–wake characteristics of the PSG.

Answer on page 149.

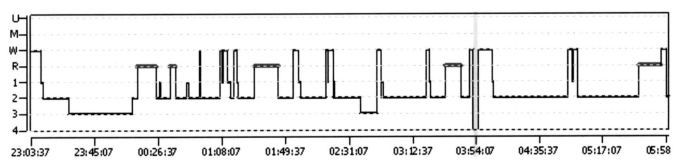

M, movement time; R, REM sleep; W, awake; 1–4, stages 1–4, respectively; time of day is reported at the bottom of the trace.

CASE 17 — A 67-year-old man with chronic sleep-onset and maintenance insomnia, as well as episodes of talking and walking in his sleep

Carl Bazil

A 67-year-old retired emergency room physician was seen for evaluation of chronic sleep-onset and maintenance insomnia, as well as episodes of talking and walking in his sleep. The latter occur nearly every night, and seem worse in times of stress. He does not report excessive daytime somnolence, and his only medication is flecainide. A representative 2 minute page of his nocturnal PSG is displayed below.

1. Based on the history and PSG interpretation, which of the following is correct?
A. The tracing shows PLMs, which could cause insomnia but not sleep-walking or sleep-talking
B. The tracing shows PLMs, which could cause sleep-walking and sleep-talking but not insomnia
C. The tracing shows PLMs, which could cause all of his symptoms
D. The tracing shows PLMs, but is likely unrelated to his insomnia
E. The tracing shows a normal PSG.

Case Studies in Polysomnography Interpretation, ed. Robert C. Basner. Published by Cambridge University Press. © Cambridge University Press 2012.

17

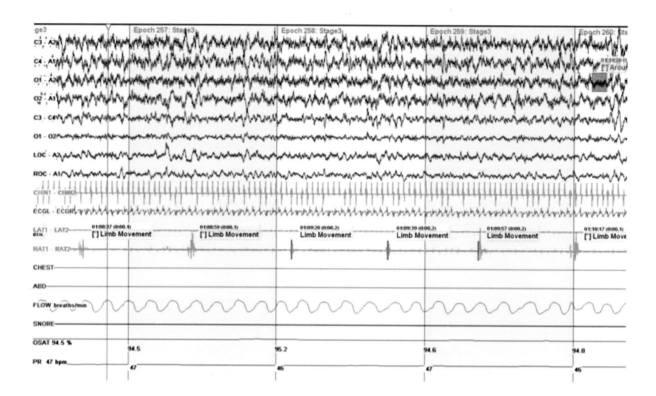

On further questioning, the patient reports that his "sleep-walking" sometimes involves kicking things such as his bedside table, and that the episodes are often associated with dream images. Dreams of shooting basketballs seem to occur relatively frequently in association with arising and moving about. The 30 second PSG tracing of REM sleep below is from the same night of study, and during this portion of the study he sat up and punched the wall at one point (not pictured here).

2. What is this PSG tracing most consistent with?

A. REM sleep without atonia
B. REM sleep with OSA
C. REM sleep with hypoventilation
D. REM sleep with artifact

Answer on page 150.

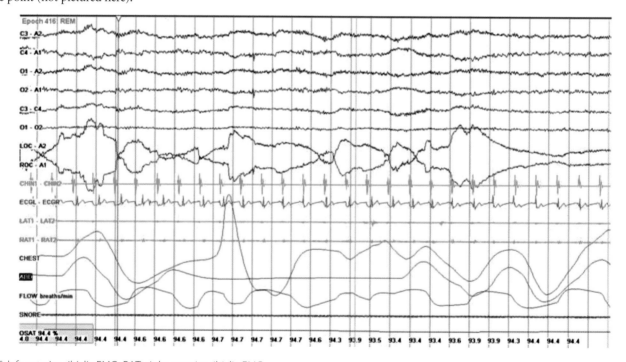

LAT, left anterior tibialis EMG; RAT, right anterior tibialis EMG.

A 77-year-old woman with sudden episodes of loss of consciousness

Carl Bazil

A 77-year-old woman was seen for sudden episodes of loss of consciousness. Although these occasionally seemed to happen without warning, most were preceded by profound sleepiness. Sleep history and medications were unremarkable, so PSG was performed. The following is a representative 2 minute tracing from this PSG.

What is the relevance of the findings on this tracing with regard to her symptoms, and what is as an appropriate treatment based on these findings?

A. Not relevant
B. Possibly relevant; consider treatment with gabapentin enacarbil
C. Possibly relevant; consider treatment with eszopiclone
D. Likely causing the symptoms; treat with gabapentin enacarbil
E. Likely causing the symptoms; treat with eszopiclone.

Answer on page 150.

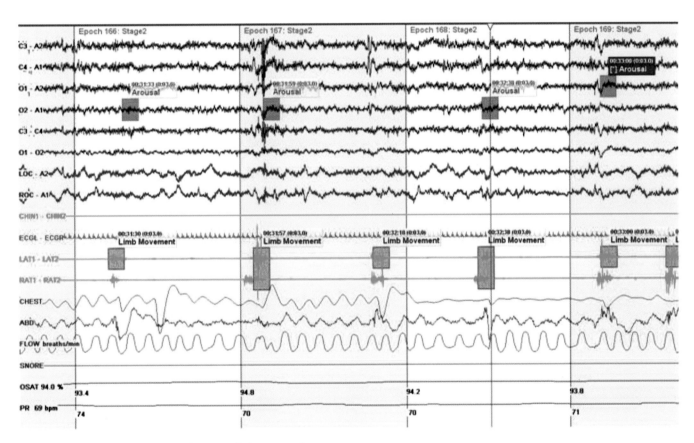

Abdomen, abdominal respiratory inductance plethysmography.

Case Studies in Polysomnography Interpretation, ed. Robert C. Basner. Published by Cambridge University Press. © Cambridge University Press 2012.

A 32-year-old woman with frequent nocturnal episodes of sudden arousal and short chaotic movements

Carl Bazil

A 32-year-old woman was evaluated for frequent nocturnal episodes of sudden arousal and chaotic movements lasting less than 30 seconds. She is immediately alert after the episodes and then usually returns to sleep. These typically occur in the first third of the night, although they have occurred at all times of sleep, including during daytime naps.

The following is a 30 second tracing from her nocturnal PSG.

What is the best interpretation of the EEG pattern at the arrow?
A. Electrographic arousal
B. Movement artifact
C. Lambda waves
D. Posterior dominant rhythm
E. Generalized spike-wave discharge.

Answer on page 151.

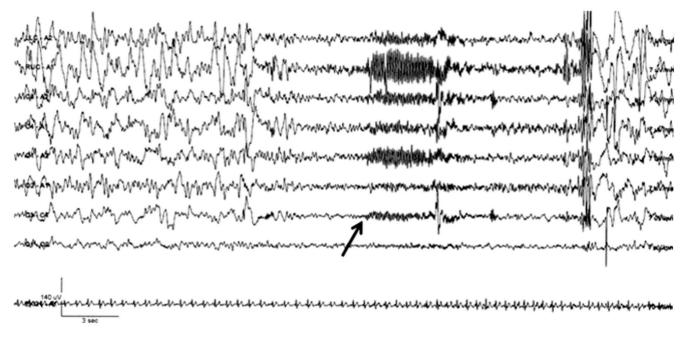

Fig. 1. LLC-A2 and RUC-A1, left and right referential EOG.

Case Studies in Polysomnography Interpretation, ed. Robert C. Basner. Published by Cambridge University Press. © Cambridge University Press 2012.

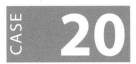

CASE 20

A 70-year-old woman with a history of hypertension and paroxysmal atrial fibrillation

Sean M. Caples

The following is a 10 second epoch from the PSG of a 70-year-old woman, showing a modified ECG lead I. The patient has a history of hypertension and paroxysmal atrial fibrillation. She is in stage N2 sleep. Heart rate is 80 bpm.

What should be the interpretation?
A. Sinus rhythm
B. Atrial fibrillation
C. Narrow complex tachycardia
D. Sinus tachycardia
E. Use a different ECG lead.

Answer on page 152.

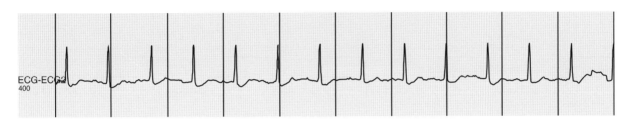

CASE 21

A 74-year-old man with known cardiac disease and an automated implantable cardioverter–defibrillator

Sean M. Caples

The following is a 30 second epoch from a nocturnal PSG displaying a modified lead I ECG. The patient is a 74-year-old man with known cardiac disease, with an automated implantable cardioverter–defibrillator in place. The patient is in stage N2 sleep throughout this tracing. The "baseline" heart rate is 70 bpm. Each vertical line is 1 second.

What is the the correct underlying cardiac rhythm identified?
A. Sinus rhythm
B. Sinus bradycardia
C. Atrial fibrillation
D. None of the above.

Answer on page 152.

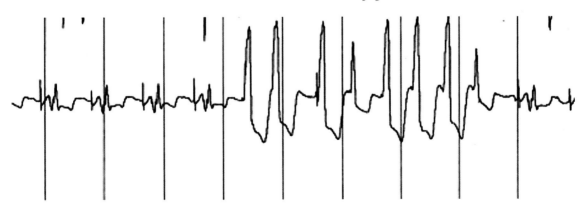

Case Studies in Polysomnography Interpretation, ed. Robert C. Basner. Published by Cambridge University Press. © Cambridge University Press 2012.

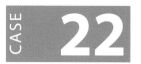

A 60-year-old man with known coronary artery disease

Sean M. Caples

The following tracing is representative of REM sleep from an overnight PSG in a 60-year-old man with known coronary artery disease undergoing study for symptoms of OSA.

What is the best interpretation of the modified lead I ECG?

A. First-degree AV block
B. Mobitz type I second-degree AV block
C. Mobitz type II second-degree AV block
D. Third-degree (complete) AV block
E. None of the above.

Answer on page 153.

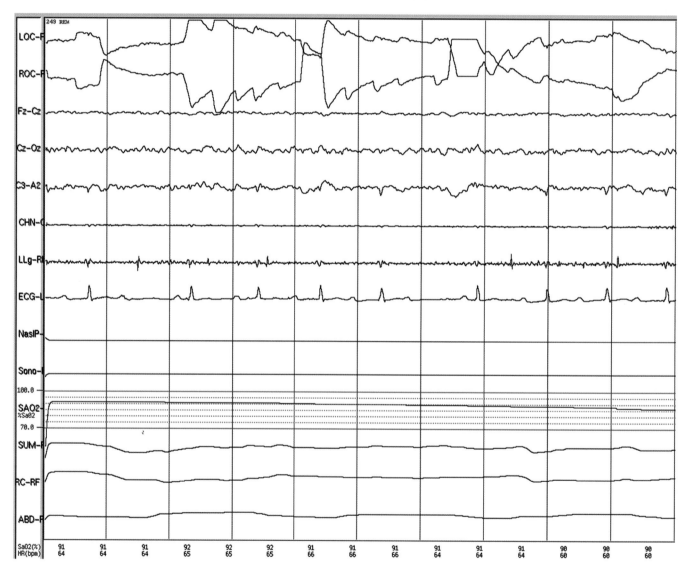

Cz-Oz, referential occipital EEG; Fz-Cz, referential frontal EEG; ECG-L, modified lead I ECG; HR, heart rate; LLg-R, left and right pretibial EMG; NasIP, nasal pressure tracing; RC-RF, thoracic respiratory effort; Sono, snore channel; SUM, summation of abdominal and thoracic respiratory inductance plethysmography.

Case Studies in Polysomnography Interpretation, ed. Robert C. Basner. Published by Cambridge University Press. © Cambridge University Press 2012.

A 38-year-old man with "restlessness" at night prior to sleep onset

Kelly A. Carden

A 38-year-old man complains of "restlessness" at night prior to sleep onset. He undergoes PSG that confirms the diagnosis of OSA. He returns to the sleep laboratory for a CPAP titration study. A 30 second representative tracing from this PSG, recorded just after lights out, is shown.

Based upon interpretation of the major abnormality seen on this tracing, what is the most accurate ICSD diagnosis?
A. Obstructive sleep apnea
B. Central sleep apnea resulting from Cheyne–Stokes breathing pattern
C. Sleep-related rhythmic movement disorder
D. Sleep-walking
E. Restless legs syndrome (RLS).

Answer on page 153.

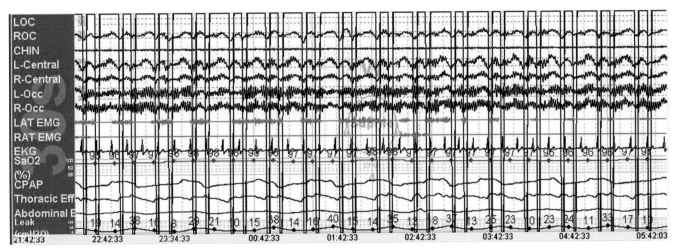

Abdominal E, abdominal respiratory inductance plethysmography; CPAP, nasal pressure at the CPAP mask; L-Central and R-central, central referential EEGs; L-Occ and R-Occ, occipital referential EEGs; Leak, leak recorded from CPAP delivery; Thoracic Eff, thoracic respiratory inductance plethysmography.

Case Studies in Polysomnography Interpretation, ed. Robert C. Basner. Published by Cambridge University Press. © Cambridge University Press 2012.

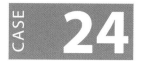

A 50-year-old previously healthy man with obstructive sleep apnea and a recent history of palpitations

Kelly A. Carden

A 50-year-old previously healthy man with OSA and a recent history of palpitations undergoes nocturnal PSG for CPAP titration. He has no other complaints prior to the PSG, but during one awakening, he complained of his heart "skipping beats."

A representative tracing (30 seconds) from his overnight PSG with CPAP is shown.

What is the best interpretation of the cardiac arrhythmia seen on the ECG?
A. Normal sinus rhythm
B. Atrial fibrillation
C. Atrial flutter
D. Ventricular bigeminy
E. Atrial bigeminy.

Answer on page 153.

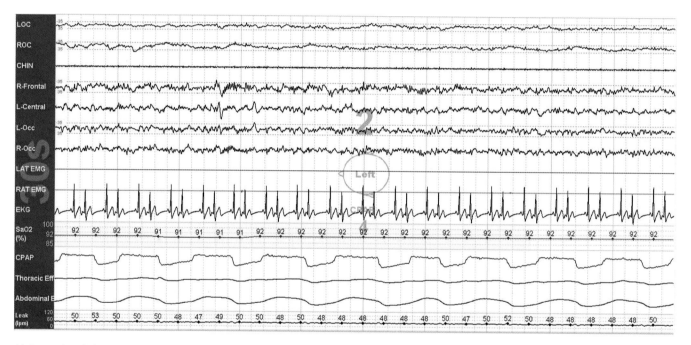

Abdominal E, abdominal respiratory inductance plethysmography; CPAP, nasal pressure at the CPAP mask; L-Central, central referential EEG; L-Occ and R-Occ, occipital referential EEGs; Leak, leak recorded from CPAP delivery; Thoracic Eff, thoracic respiratory inductance plethysmography.

Case Studies in Polysomnography Interpretation, ed. Robert C. Basner. Published by Cambridge University Press. © Cambridge University Press 2012.

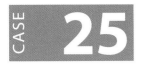
A 53-year-old man with a history of loud snoring and daytime sleepiness

Kelly A. Carden

A 53-year-old man with a history of loud snoring and daytime sleepiness is referred for a PSG to rule out OSA.

A representative 2 minute tracing from his overnight diagnostic PSG is shown.

Which of the following best describes the respiratory event seen in the tracing?

A. Obstructive apnea
B. Central apnea
C. Obstructive hypopnea
D. A non-pathologic event
E. A pathologic event that was not scored by the technologist.

Answer on page 154.

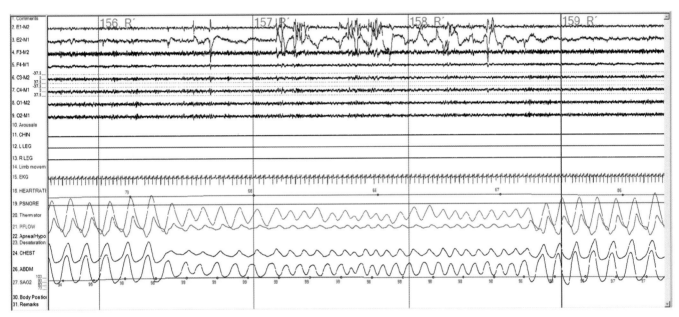

Apnea/hypo, scored respiratory events (by AASM criteria); Arousals, scored arousals; Body position and remarks, comments from technologist about position/other findings; Desaturation, scored desaturations of 3% or greater; F3-M2, left frontal EEG; F4-M2, right frontal EEG; Limb movem, scored PLMs; PFlow, nasal air pressure transducer.

A 27-year-old man with a 10 year history of insomnia

Kelly A. Carden

A 27-year-old man presents complaining of a 10 year history of insomnia. He reports primarily sleep-onset insomnia, indicating that he is not sleepy until "the middle of the night." He denies any precipitating factor or history of shift work. His sleep-onset latency is reported to be between 2 and 3 hours. He reports "I am only functional because I catch up when I can." He has tried three different hypnotics and melatonin (all prescribed by his primary care physician to be taken within 30 minutes of goal bedtime), but still has trouble falling asleep.

Figure 1 is a typical actigraphy tracing from this patient, but note that one of the sleep opportunites on each day was highlighted by the clinician for effect when describing the results to the patient (banner above the tracing). Also note that this is a double plot actigraphy tracing where the data are presented twice (see the circles as an example, look at the patterns for similarities). The time legend also helps to make the determination of single versus double plotting as there are two of each time point. For example, there are two "04" time points, which both correspond to 04:00 (refer to the arrows).

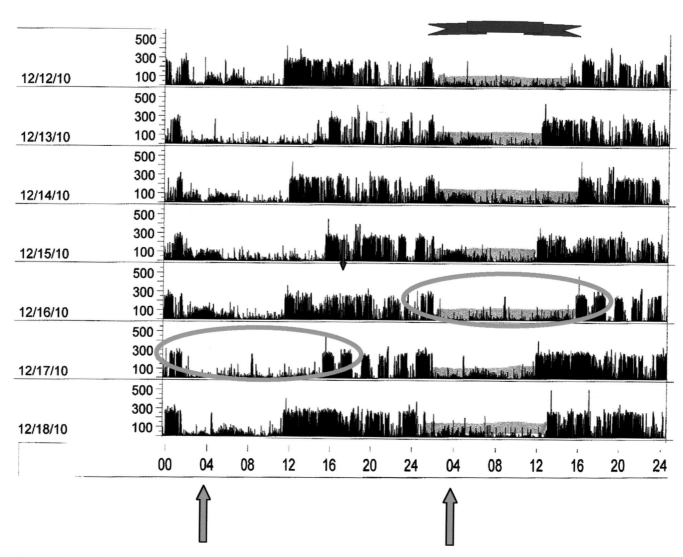

Fig. 1. Green circles indicate an example of repeated data; blue banner above the tracing outlines a sleep opportunity.

Case Studies in Polysomnography Interpretation, ed. Robert C. Basner. Published by Cambridge University Press. © Cambridge University Press 2012.

1. **Which one of the following is *not* accurate regarding the actigraphy tracing?**
   A. The bedtime is relatively consistent and is at midnight or later
   B. The sleep-onset latency is variable
   C. The time in bed is variable
   D. The out of bed time is variable
   E. Once asleep, he does not have maintenance insomnia.

2. **What is the most likely diagnosis based on the above history and interpretation of the actigraphy tracing?**
   A. Advanced sleep phase syndrome
   B. Delayed sleep phase syndrome
   C. Non-24 hour sleep–wake syndrome
   D. Jet lag sleep disorder
   E. Circadian rhythm disorder, irregular sleep–wake type.

   Answer on page 154.

Figure 2 indicates bedtime and out of bed time.

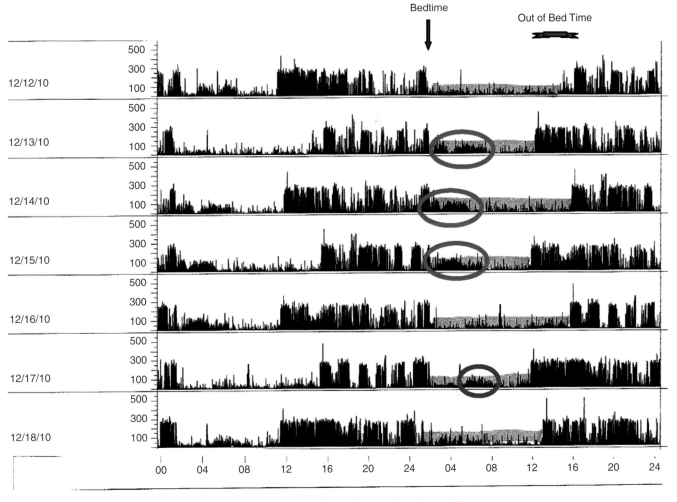

Fig. 2. Blue circles indicate wake time after onset of sleep; red circles indicate activity after bedtime.

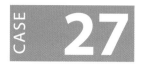

A patient's sleeping habits shown in an actigraph

Kelly A. Carden

The following is a 7 day actigraphy tracing in a patient.

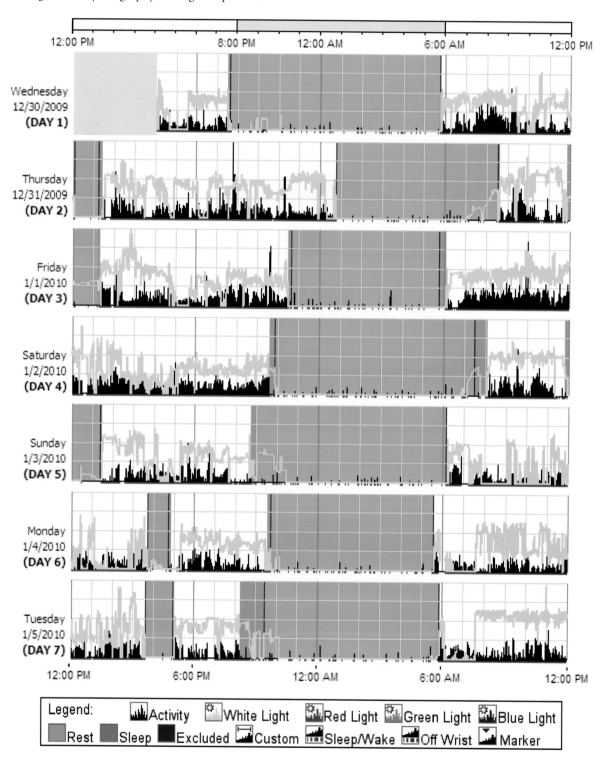

Case Studies in Polysomnography Interpretation, ed. Robert C. Basner. Published by Cambridge University Press. © Cambridge University Press 2012.

Which one of the following is incorrect regarding the actigraphy shown in the above tracing?
A. The patient sleeps more than 8.5 hours per day on average
B. The patient takes naps
C. The actigraphy monitor used for this study also has white light monitoring technology

D. The actigraphy tracing is a double plot tracing (as opposed to a single plot)
E. The patient's bedtimes and wake times are variable.

Answer on page 155.

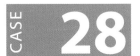

A patient with a possible sleep-related breathing disorder

Christopher Cielo and Lee J. Brooks

A patient was referred for a possible sleep-related breathing disorder. The overnight PSG tracing below was obtained.

What is the best interpretation of the findings?
A. Abrupt discontinuation of fluoxetine
B. No sleep for 36 hours prior to recording
C. Narcolepsy
D. Hypnogram of a four-month-old child
E. Cocaine withdrawal.

Answer on page 155.

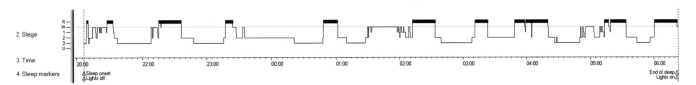

R, REM sleep; W, awake; 1, N1 sleep; 2, N2 sleep; 3, N3 sleep.

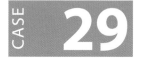

CASE 29

A 4-month-old boy with a history of prematurity, gastroesophageal reflux, and observed pauses in breathing during sleep

Christopher Cielo and Lee J. Brooks

A 4-month-old boy with a history of prematurity and gastro-esophageal reflux was referred for overnight PSG to investigate observed pauses in breathing during sleep.

What respiratory finding(s) are seen in this 60 second tracing?

A. Obstructive sleep apnea
B. Four central apneas
C. Periodic breathing sequence
D. No respiratory events
E. Upper airway resistance syndrome.

Answer on page 156.

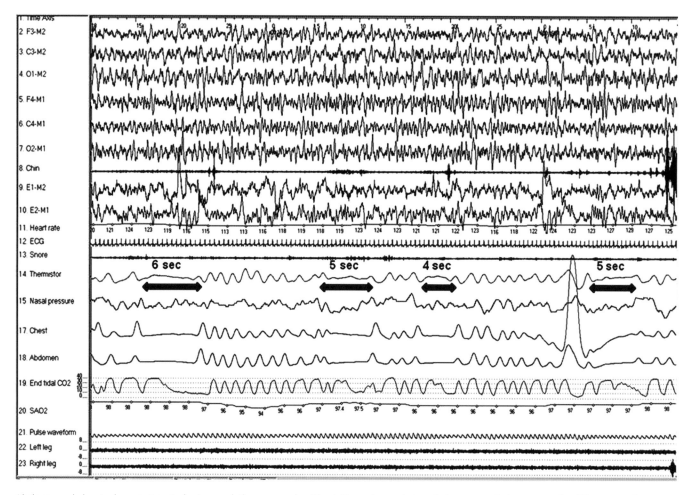

Abdomen, abdominal respiratory inductance plethysmography; Chest, thoracic respiratory inductance plethysmography; ETco$_2$, waveform derived from continuous CO$_2$ measurement; Left leg, left leg EMG; Nasal pressure, nasal pressure transducer; Right leg, right leg EMG time axis, seconds.

Case Studies in Polysomnography Interpretation, ed. Robert C. Basner. Published by Cambridge University Press. © Cambridge University Press 2012.

A 7-day-old female with Pierre–Robin sequence and micrognathia

Christopher Cielo and Carole L. Marcus

A 7-day-old female with Pierre–Robin sequence and micrognathia was referred for PSG by the neonatologist to assess O_2 desaturations during sleep. The following 30 second epoch was captured from the overnight PSG. Baseline O_2 saturation was low as a result of a respiratory event prior to this epoch.

What is the correct interpretation of the respiratory event seen in this epoch?

A. No abnormal respiratory event
B. Obstructive apnea
C. Hypopnea
D. Central apnea
E. Mixed apnea.

Answer on page 156.

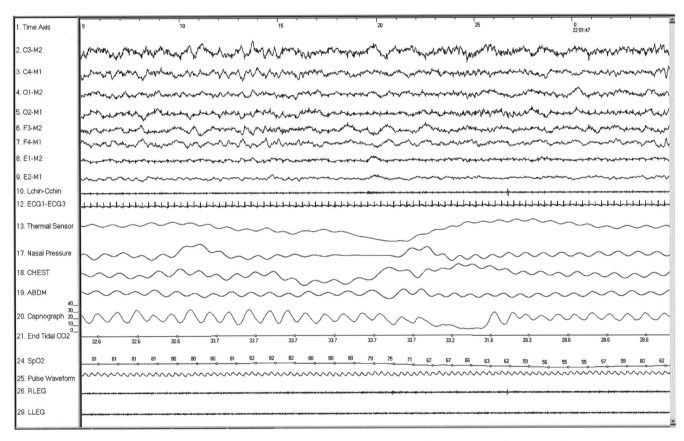

Capnograph, waveform derived from continuous CO_2 measurement; Nasal pressure, nasal pressure transducer; time axis, seconds; Spo_2 by pusle oximetry.

A 3-year-old girl with a history of static encephalopathy and severe obstructive sleep apnea

Christopher Cielo and Carole L. Marcus

A 3-year-old girl with a history of static encephalopathy and severe OSA was referred to the sleep laboratory for PAP titration. The study began on CPAP, but the patient was switched to bilevel pressure of 10 cmH$_2$O IPAP and 5 cmH$_2$O EPAP in the spontaneous timed mode, with a rate of 14 breaths/min, because of her central apneas. A 60 second tracing is shown.

What is the best interpretation of the respiratory findings on this 60 second tracing?

A. The patient continues to have obstructive apnea because of insufficient EPAP

B. The machine is not triggering the patient's chest wall to rise

C. The mechanical ventilation is set at a supraphysiologic rate

D. The patient continues to have hypopnea because of insufficient EPAP.

Answer on page 157.

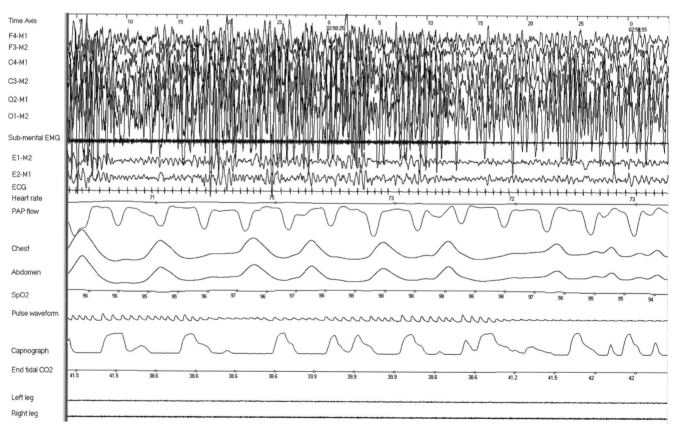

Abdomen, abdominal respiratory inductance plethysmography; Capnograph, waveform derived from continuous CO$_2$ measurement; Left leg, left leg EMG; PAP flow, airflow derived from pressure signal; Right leg, right leg EMG; time axis, seconds.

Case Studies in Polysomnography Interpretation, ed. Robert C. Basner. Published by Cambridge University Press. © Cambridge University Press 2012.

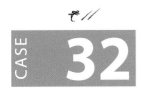
32 A 63-year-old woman with non-apneic oxyhemoglobin desaturation

David G. Davila, Patti Reed, and B. Marshall

A 63-year-old woman presented on referral from her pulmonologist for possible OSA. She reported a history of snoring and possible pauses in breathing as reported by her husband. Her primary care physician had placed her on 4 L/min O_2 through a nasal cannula both awake and asleep. Her Epworth Sleepiness Scale score was 9/24.

Her past medical history was significant for systemic hypertension, being treated with amlodipine; COPD, treated with albuterol, ipratropium, Proair, and prednisone; diabetes mellitus, treated with metformin and glyburide (glibenclamide); and depression, treated with citalopram. She is surgically menopausal but not on hormone replacement.

The patient underwent attended PSG and was found to be a simple snorer with an AHI of 2.1. It appeared that the patient was hypoventilating in sleep in a non-apneic fashion,

with prolonged and progressive desaturations noted to 81% amidst fairly well-preserved thermistor flow, nasal cannula pressure, chest and abdominal effort signals, as seen in the compressed PSG tracing (Fig. 1, displayed nadir Spo_2 in this tracing is 83%).

At PSG, arterial blood gases were obtained awake breathing room air and asleep breathing supplemental O_2 as follows:

awake room air: pH 7.38, Pco_2 59 mmHg, Po_2 42 mmHg
asleep 1 L/min O_2: pH 7.37, Pco_2 68 mmHg, Po_2 59 mmHg
asleep 3 L/min O_2: pH 7.33, Pco_2 71 mmHg, Po_2 92 mmHg.

Hypoventilation was present awake, with Pco_2 of 59 mmHg. By AASM definition, hypoventilation was present asleep with Pco_2 increasing more than 10 mmHg from awake (59 to 71 mmHg), which confirmed the interpretation of the raw breathing signals.

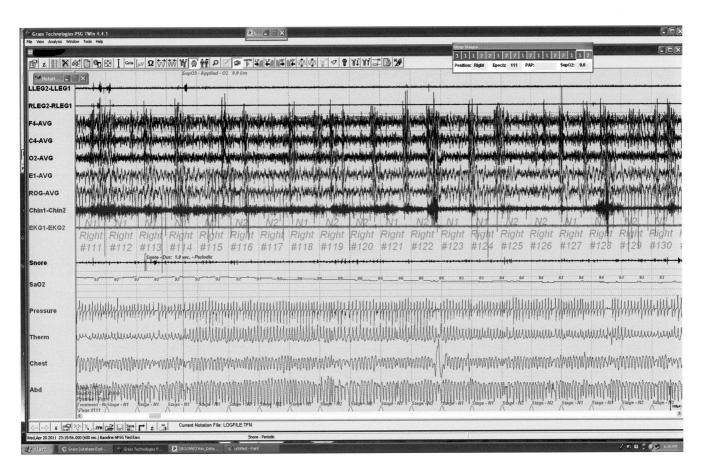

Fig. 1. Therm, oral-nasal thermistor; Spo_2 from pulse oximetry.

Case Studies in Polysomnography Interpretation, ed. Robert C. Basner. Published by Cambridge University Press. © Cambridge University Press 2012.

Subsequent SpO_2 recordings at home on supplemental O_2 showed persistent oxyhemoglobin desaturation in sleep, as displayed in Figs. 2 and 3.

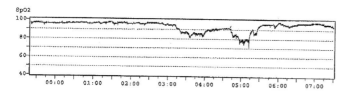

Fig. 2. SpO_2 trace on 2 L/min O_2 in sleep at home with $>$ 41 min of O_2 desaturation $\leqslant$ 88%

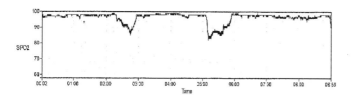

Fig. 3. SpO_2 trace on 3 L/min O_2 in sleep at home with $>$ 14 minutes of O_2 desaturation $\leqslant$ 88%

On review of the US Center for Medicare and Medicaid Services (CMS)[1] for consideration of adding non-invasive PAP, it was noted that the patient fulfilled the following criteria for COPD.

1. Diagnosis of COPD: pulmonologist diagnosed her with COPD by signs, symptoms, smoking history and PFTs (FEV1 0.48 L, and FVC 1.19 L).
2. Sleep oximetry showing $\geqslant$ 5 minutes of desaturation on 2 L/min O_2 or patient's usual fraction of inspired oxygen (FiO_2): patient's oximetry recordings on both 2 and 3 L/min O_2 showed $\geqslant$ 5 minutes of desaturation in sleep at home.
3. $PcO_2 \geqslant$ 52 mmHg awake on usual FiO_2: patient's awake PcO_2 was elevated, at 59 mmHg.

OSA was considered in the initial diagnostic differential but was ruled out on PSG: CPAP was considered but ruled out as a treatment option because of the non-apneic desaturation mechanism, as seen on the representative PSG in Fig. 1.

The patient then underwent attended PSG for a bilevel PAP (BPAP) titration. It was found that BPAP at 22/8 cmH_2O IPAP/EPAP with 1–2 L/min O_2 in-line was able to improve O_2 desaturations in sleep better than O_2 alone.

The patient reported less dyspnea at night on BPAP plus O_2 at home compared with O_2 alone, and had improved sleep

quality. A follow-up oximetry recording on BPAP and O_2 was obtained (Fig. 4).

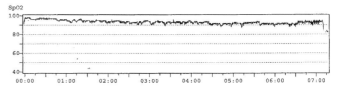

Fig. 4. SpO_2 on BPAP S (spontaneous) 22/8 cmH_2O IPAP/EPAP with 1–2 L/min O_2 in-line at home.

The patient reported quick adaptation to BPAP plus O_2 at home with nightly use. A download of adherence data obtained at about 1 month on therapy showed a stable pattern of use, with 80% of nights having $\geqslant$ 4 hours of use per night, satisfying CMS coverage criteria for BPAP (Fig. 5)

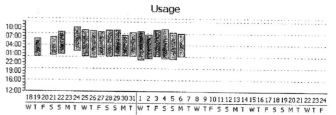

Fig. 5.

Arterial blood gases were obtained after about 1 month of using this therapy for sleep. At 9 a.m. breathing room air, the following was obtained: pH 7.42, PcO_2 55 mmHg, and PO_2 52 mmHg.

1. **Which of the following is true in regard to nocturnal or sleep-related oxyhemoglobin desaturation in patients with COPD?**
   A. Occurs only if OSA is present
   B. Oxygen alone is needed for treatment
   C. Bilevel PAP alone is needed for treatment
   D. None of the above.

2. **What is required under the CMS criteria, to qualify a patient with COPD for BPAP during sleep?**
   A. Little, it is easy
   B. that OSA is ruled out
   C. that the patient desaturates in sleep
   D. None of the above.

Answer on page 157.

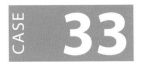

A 24-year-old woman with a history of anxiety, asthma, and daytime sleepiness

Katherine A. Dudley and Jean K. Matheson

A 24-year-old woman with a history of anxiety and asthma presented for evaluation of daytime sleepiness. She complained of extreme difficulty awakening in the morning at 6 a.m. for her job as a teacher despite a typical sleep-onset time of 8:00 p.m. On weekends, she reported sleeping later but never feeling rested. She complained of an overwhelming urge to sleep during the day, with non-restorative napping. Medications included paroxetine and an oral contraceptive. Past medical, social, and family history were unremarkable, as were review of systems and physical examination.

Sleep history revealed no reported snoring, witnessed apneas, restless legs or PLMs, parasomnia-like behavior, cataplexy, sleep paralysis, or hypnagogic hallucinations. Her Epworth Sleepiness Scale score was 21/24.

Sleep logs obtained for 2 weeks prior to the PSG study revealed frequent napping in the late afternoon in addition to a regular sleep period between 8 p.m. and 6 a.m. during the work week. During weekends, her sleep onset was 9 to 10 p.m., wake time was close to 9:00 a.m., and she demonstrated more frequent daytime napping.

After discontinuing medications for several weeks, she completed an overnight PSG study and an MSLT on the following day, with hypnograms shown below.

Based on this history and interpretation of these sleep study hypnograms, what is the most likely diagnosis?
A. Narcolepsy without cataplexy
B. Idiopathic hypersomnia
C. Behaviorally induced insufficient sleep syndrome
D. Delayed sleep phase disorder
E. Narcolepsy with cataplexy.

Answer on page 158.

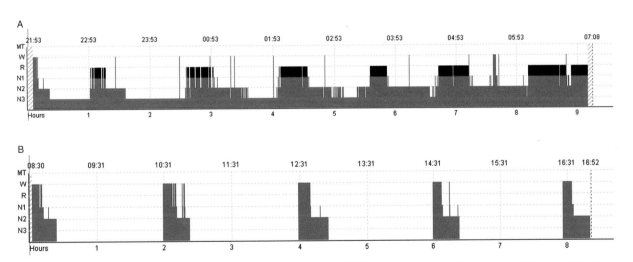

(A) Hypnogram of overnight PSG; (B) MSLT hypnogram. MT, movement time; R, REM (with black bars); W, stage wake; N1, stage N1; N2, stage N2; N3, stage N3; *x* axis, time (clock time above, hours after lights out below).

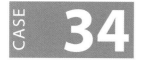

CASE 34

A 43-year-old Chinese man with a history of obesity, difficult-to-control hypertension, and proteinuria, with daytime sleepiness and snoring

Katherine A. Dudley and Robert Thomas

A 43-year-old Chinese man with a history of obesity, difficult-to-control hypertension, and proteinuria is referred to the sleep clinic for evaluation, given his daytime sleepiness and snoring. Sleep timing is consistently 12:00 a.m. until 9:00 a.m., after the patient finishes his job working in a restaurant. He reports feeling tired and sleepy during the course of the day, particularly late in the afternoon. Sleeping longer has not relieved the symptoms. Physical examination is remarkable for hypertension (145/90 mmHg), crowded oropharynx, and obesity. He is only taking antihypertensive drugs.

The patient is sent for a PSG evaluation and a diagnostic portion is shown in Fig. 1. Figure 2 shows the associated hypnogram.

Based on the displayed diagnostic portion of his PSG and hypnogram, how is the patient's sleep-disordered breathing pathology best characterized?

A. Obstructive sleep apnea, REM dominant
B. Periodic breathing
C. Primary obstructive pathology, with secondary chemoreceptor sensitization
D. Cheyne–Stokes breathing.

Answer on page 159.

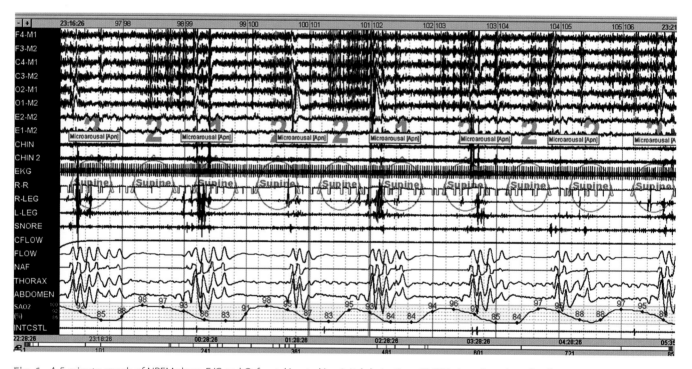

Fig. 1. A 5 minute epoch of NREM sleep; F/C and O, frontal/central/occipital derivations; FLOW, thermistor-based airflow; M, mastoid; NAF, nasal pressure tranducer.

Case Studies in Polysomnography Interpretation, ed. Robert C. Basner. Published by Cambridge University Press. © Cambridge University Press 2012.

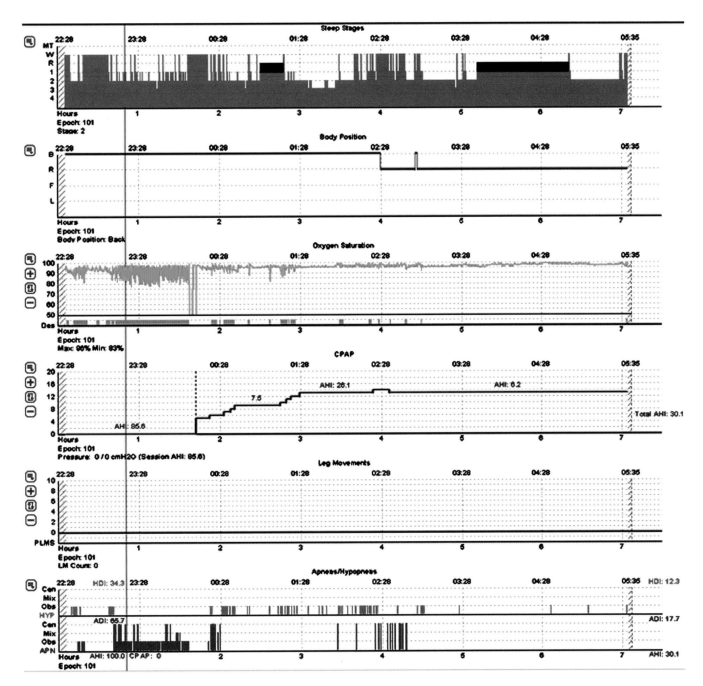

Fig. 2. Extended hypnogram, from top: sleep stages, body position, oximetry, PAP, motor activation (legs) and respiratory scoring tags.

A 57-year-old man with a history of mild dyslipidemia who had a cerebrovascular accident several months earlier

Katherine A. Dudley and Robert Thomas

A 57-year-old man with a history of mild dyslipidemia presents to the sleep clinic. Several months before, he had suffered a cerebrovascular accident, experiencing right hand numbness and weakness. Magnetic resonance imaging (MRI) demonstrated a small infarct to the left frontal area. Extensive work-up, including Holter monitoring, transthoracic and transesophageal echocardiogram, lower extremity duplex scan, and hypercoagulable state work-up was unrevealing. It was not felt that mild dyslipidemia alone was a likely explanation for his cerebrovascular accident, given his overall good health and healthy lifestyle. A PSG was sought to determine whether sleep-disordered breathing could have been a risk factor for the cerebrovascular accident. A fragment of the diagnostic study is shown in Fig. 1. The patient then returned for a CPAP titration study, with a fragment of this titration study shown in Fig. 2 and a 5 minute window from later that night in Fig. 3.

What does the PAP titration study demonstrate?
A. Normal transient habituation effect with PAP
B. Normal central apnea in REM at time of sleep onset
C. Central apnea induced by CPAP (traditionally defined complex sleep apnea)
D. Central apnea secondary to the cerebrovascular accident, with Cheyne–Stokes breathing.

Answer on page 160.

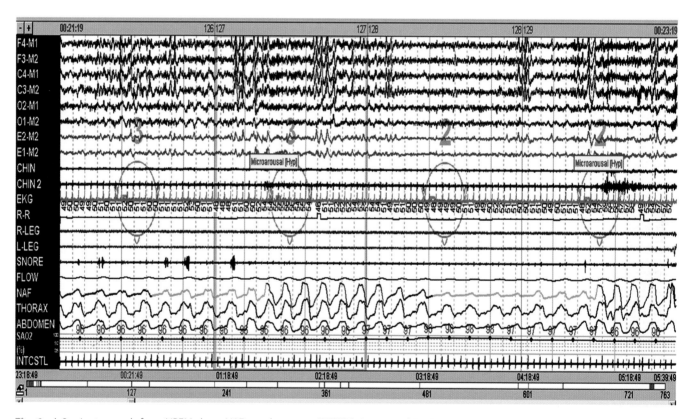

Fig. 1. A 2 minute epoch from NREM sleep. NAF, nasal pressure; INTCSTL, intercostal EMG; SAO2, O₂ saturation from pulse oximetry.

Case Studies in Polysomnography Interpretation, ed. Robert C. Basner. Published by Cambridge University Press. © Cambridge University Press 2012.

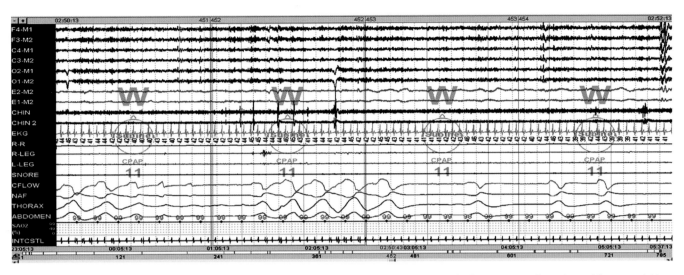

Fig. 2. A 2 minute epoch from NREM sleep. Channels are the same as in Fig. 1 except CFLOW, which is a PAP machine derived flow signal. Note the central apneas; these occurred at virtually every pressure tested.

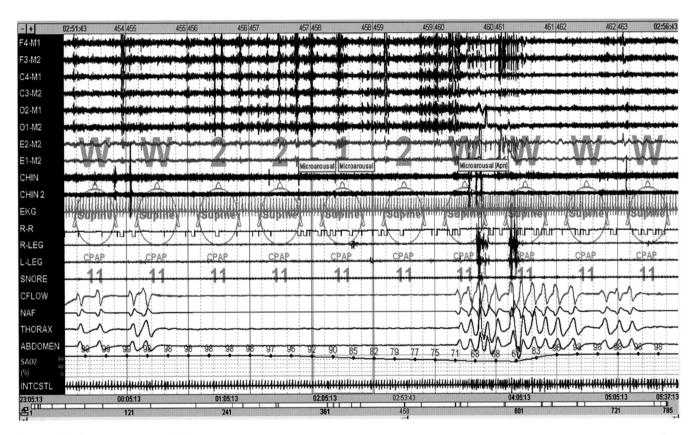

Fig. 3. A 5 minute epoch from NREM sleep.

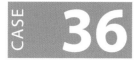
A 29-year-old man who is mildly overweight, with a history of depression and attention deficit hyperactivity disorder, with difficulty falling asleep and daytime sleepiness

Katherine A. Dudley and Robert Thomas

A 29-year-old man who is mildly overweight, with a history of depression and attention deficit hyperactivity disorder, presents to the sleep clinic with difficulty falling asleep and daytime sleepiness. His sleep history is notable for attempting to go to bed around 11:00 p.m. or midnight, and remaining awake until closer to 3 or 4:00 a.m. He often plays video games or uses his laptop if he cannot sleep or feels anxious. His wife reports loud snoring and witnessed apneas.

After working on management of his circadian phase with melatonin and light, and improving sleep hygiene, his sleep initiation insomnia has improved; however, he says he still has continued daytime sleepiness and a sense of non-restorative sleep.

He undergoes an overnight PSG study, with two fragments shown below.

Based upon interpretation of these PSG tracings, and the history, what should be recommended as the next step in his management and/or evaluation?
A. Undergo a CPAP titration study
B. Head MRI
C. Hypnotic medication
D. Weight loss.

Answer on page 161.

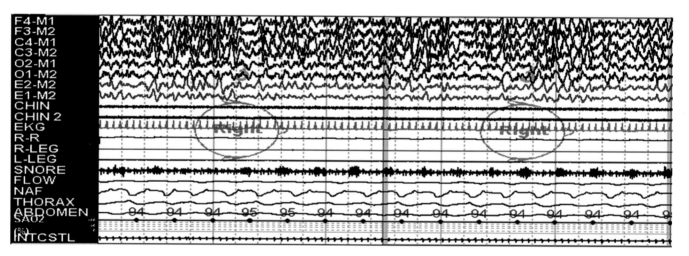

Fig. 1. NREM sleep. Vertical thin green lines every 15 seconds.

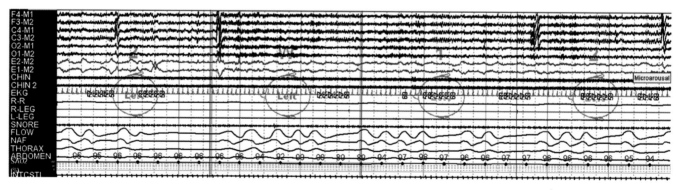

Fig. 2. A 3 minute epoch from NREM sleep.

Case Studies in Polysomnography Interpretation, ed. Robert C. Basner. Published by Cambridge University Press. © Cambridge University Press 2012.

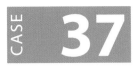

The following is a 30 second epoch from a PSG.

From what part of the brain is the finding marked with the arrow generated?
A. Lateral and posterior portions of the hypothalamus
B. Locus coeruleus
C. Thalamic reticular nuclei
D. Pineal gland
E. Tuberomammillary nucleus.

Answer on page 161.

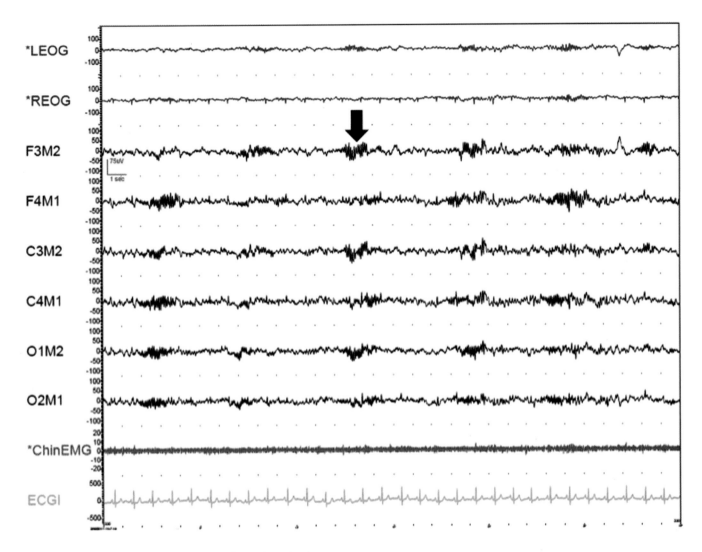

LEOG, left referential eye lead; REOG, right referential eye lead.

Case Studies in Polysomnography Interpretation, ed. Robert C. Basner. Published by Cambridge University Press. © Cambridge University Press 2012.

A 29-year-old man assessed for a diagnosis of narcolepsy

Neil Freedman

A 29-year-old man is undergoing an MSLT as part of a work-up to support a diagnosis of narcolepsy. During the first nap trial of the MSLT, the patient achieves stage N1 sleep 4 minutes into the trial and the study is permitted to continue after the initial sleep onset. The tracings show four 30 second epochs (A–D).

Based on this information and interpretation of the MSLT tracings, the MSLT should be terminated after which one of the following four 30 second epochs (A–D)?

Answer on page 162.

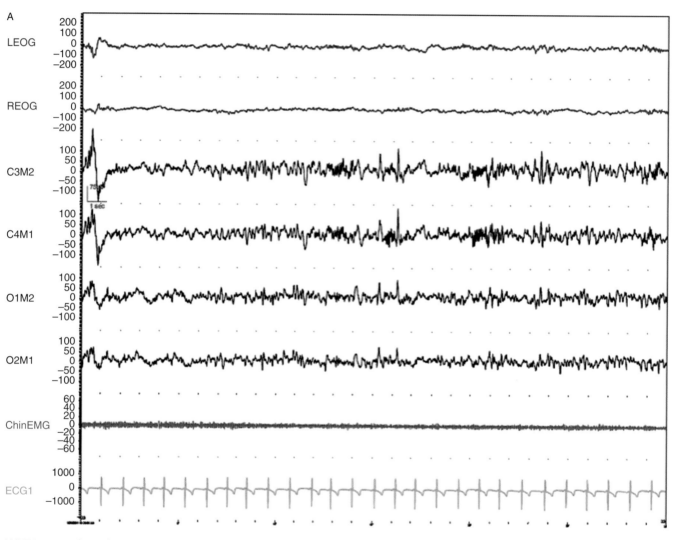

MSLT 30 second epoch A.

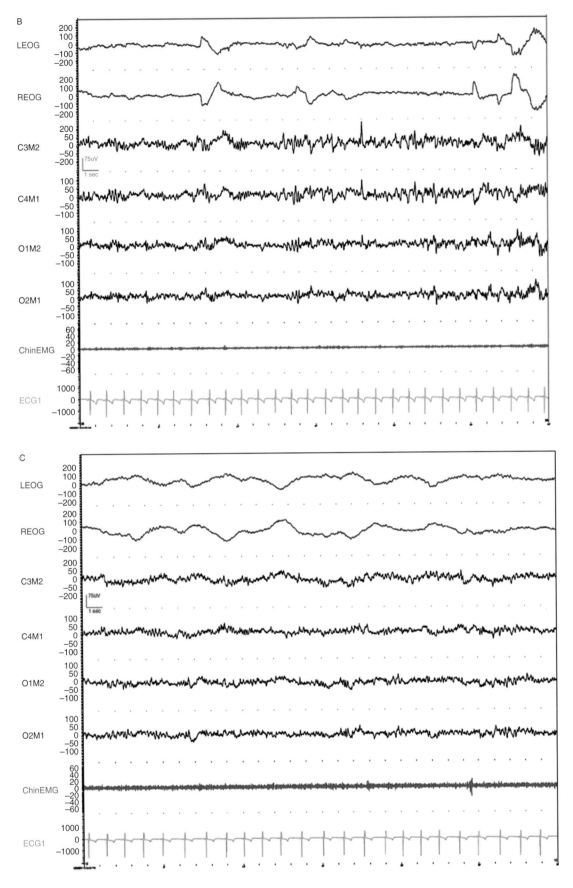

MSLT 30 second epochs B–C.

D

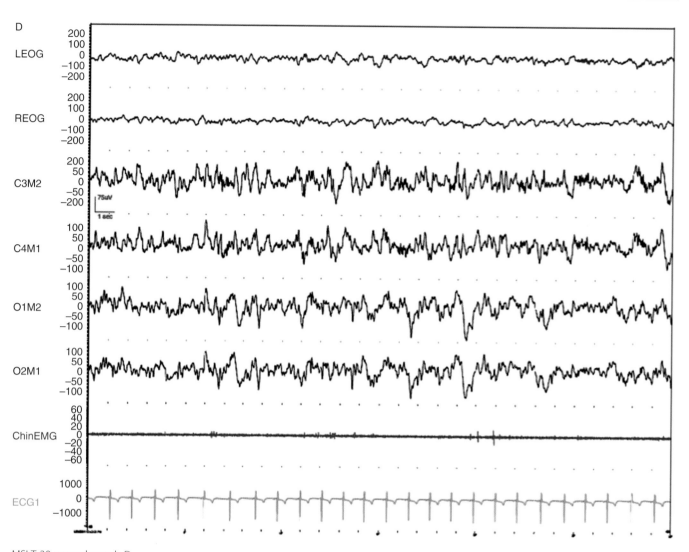

MSLT 30 second epoch D.

A 24-year-old man with symptoms of excessive daytime sleepiness

Neil Freedman

A 24-year-old man presents with symptoms of excessive daytime sleepiness (Epworth Sleepiness Scale score, 15/24) over the last several years. He denies cataplexy, RLS symptoms, a history of head trauma, or snoring. He takes no medications, has no previous medical problems and has a normal physical examination. He undergoes a five nap MSLT with the following results.

Based on this clinical presentation, the MSLT hypnogram and the summarized results, what recommendation should be made?

A. Initiate sodium oxybate
B. Initiate modafinil
C. Titration with CPAP
D. None of the above; there are insufficient data to decide.

Answer on page 162.

A

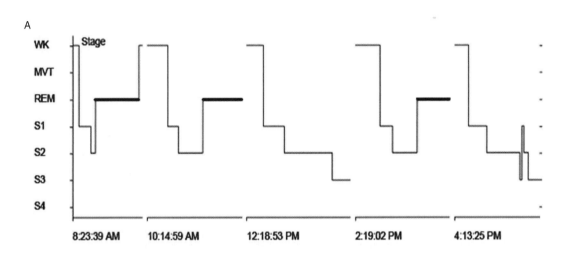

B

	Nap 1	Nap 2	Nap 3	Nap 4	Nap 5
Lights OFF	8:23:39 AM	10:14:59 AM	12:18:53 PM	2:19:02 PM	4:13:25 PM
Sleep onset (SO)	8:25:09 AM	10:19:59 AM	12:22:53 PM	2:25:02 PM	4:16:55 PM
Lights ON	8:40:39 AM	10:37:59 AM	12:43:53 PM	2:42:02 PM	4:34:25 PM
Time in Bed	17'00"	23'00"	25'00"	23'00"	21'00"
Tot Sleep Time	14'30"	18'00"	21'00"	17'00"	17'30"
Sleep latency	01'30"	05'00"	04'00"	06'00"	03'30"
REM latency	04'00"	08'30"	/	09'00"	/

Average sleep latency (5 values) : 04'00"
Average REM latency (3 values) : 07'10"

(A) Hypnograms from five consecutive MSLT nap trials. Sleep stages are represented on vertical axis and individual MSLT nap start times are represented on the horizontal axis. (B) Data from the individual nap trials. The average sleep latency represents the mean sleep latency.

A 43-year-old obese man with a history of snoring

Neil Freedman

A 43-year-old man with a history of snoring and a BMI of 33kg/m^2 undergoes a routine PSG for suspected OSA. Upon reviewing the study the next day, the technician reports a "sensor malfunction" that occurred throughout the entire study. The following 2 minute epoch is representative of the data collection from the study.

Based on this tracing and the history, what would be expected to be seen this study?

A. Underestimation of the number of apneas
B. Overestimation of the arousal index
C. Underestimation of the number of hypopneas
D. Overestimation of the AHI.

Answer on page 163.

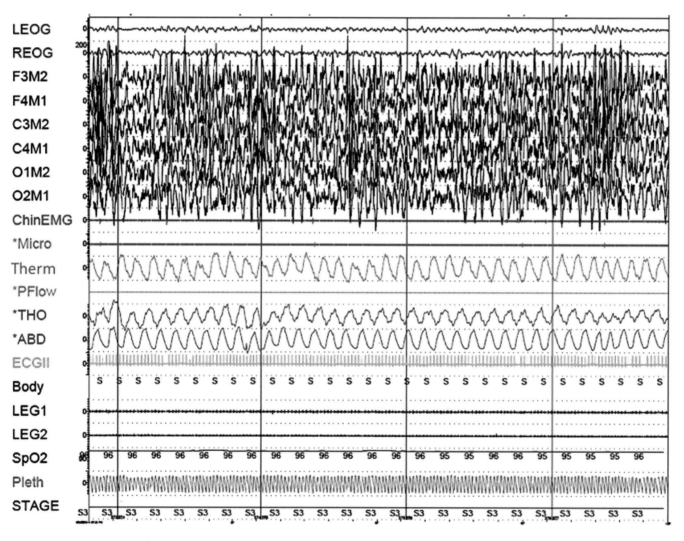

Body, body position; Leg1, tibial EMG; Leg2, tibial EMG; Micro, snore channel; Stage, sleep stage.

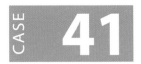

A maintenance of wakefulness test

Neil Freedman

The tracings show four 30 second epochs (A–D) from an MWT.

After which one of the epochs (A–D) should the trial be terminated?

Answer on page 163.

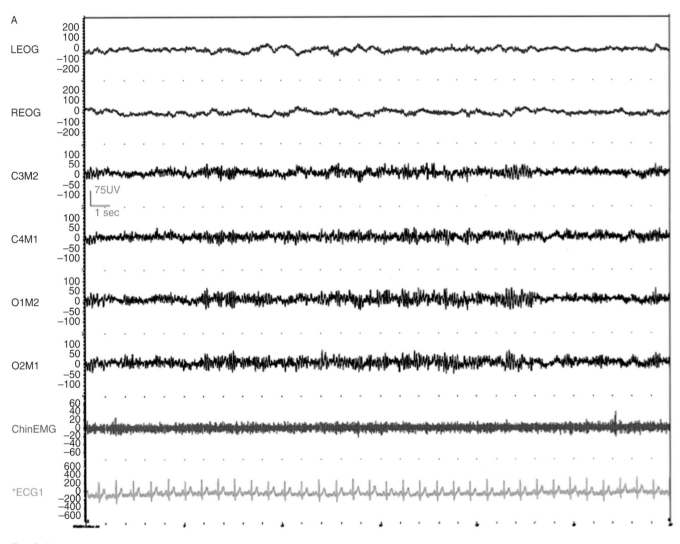

Epoch A.

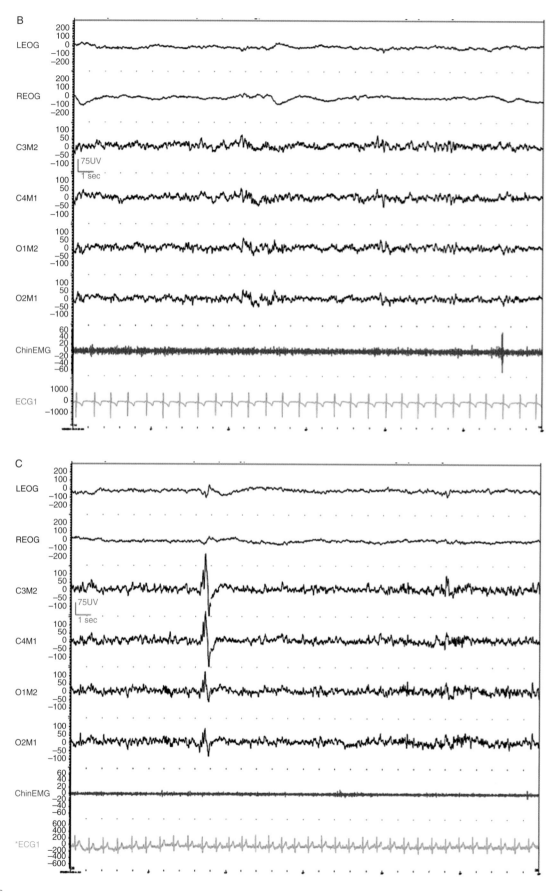

Epochs B–C.

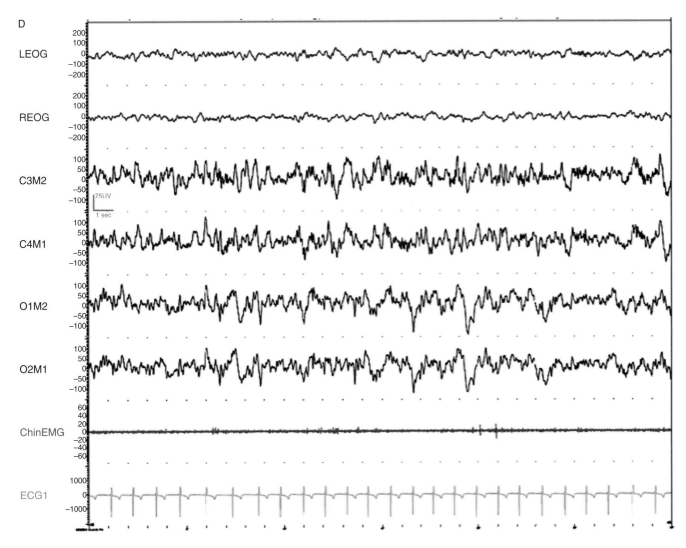

Epoch D.

The following is a PSG tracing of a sleep stage.

Which one of the following statements is correct regarding the sleep stage shown in the tracing?

A. The release of growth hormone is associated with its onset
B. It is more prevalent in the second half of the nocturnal sleep period

C. Circadian processes mediate its timing and duration
D. Compared with children, individuals over the age of 60 years have more of this sleep stage
E. It is suppressed by tricyclic antidepressants.

Answer on page 164.

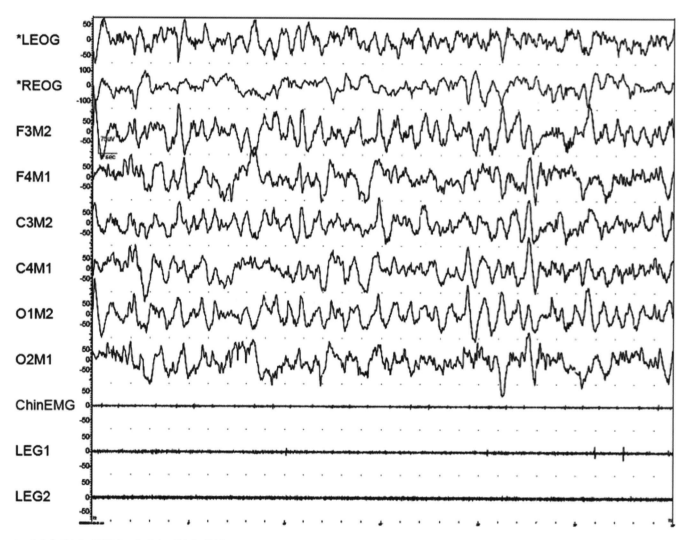

Leg1, left tibialis EMG; Leg2, right tibialis EMG.

Case Studies in Polysomnography Interpretation, ed. Robert C. Basner. Published by Cambridge University Press. © Cambridge University Press 2012.

43 Analysis of a precordial electrocardiogram finding

Neil Freedman

A 6 second ECG trace from a PSG is shown.

This precordial ECG finding is associated with which one of the following?
A. Increased incidence in patients with OSA
B. Decreased prevalence with increasing age

C. Consistent resolution with CPAP treatment in patients with OSA
D. Reduced mortality in patients with congestive heart failure.

Answer on page 164.

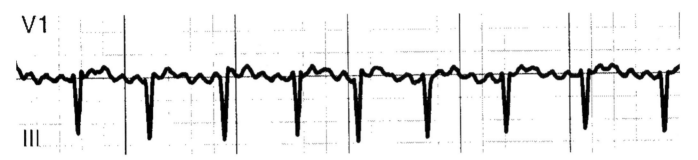

Each solid vertical line represents 1 second.

44 Linkage of episodes of gastroesophageal reflux with polysomnogram epochs

Neil Freedman

Four 30 second epochs from a PSG of a patient with gastro-esophageal reflux are displayed.

During which of the following epochs (A–D) are episodes of gastroesophageal reflux most likely to occur?

Answer on page 165.

Case Studies in Polysomnography Interpretation, ed. Robert C. Basner. Published by Cambridge University Press. © Cambridge University Press 2012.

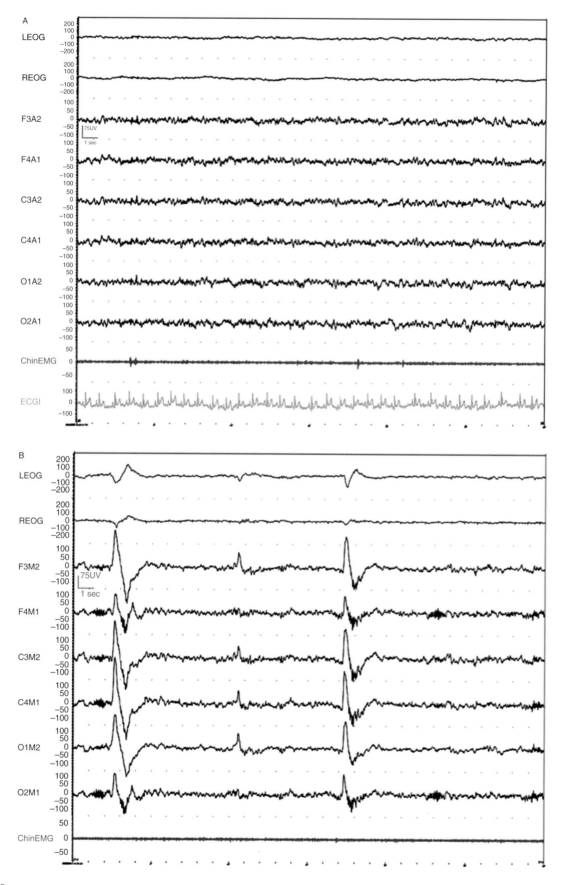

Epochs A–B.

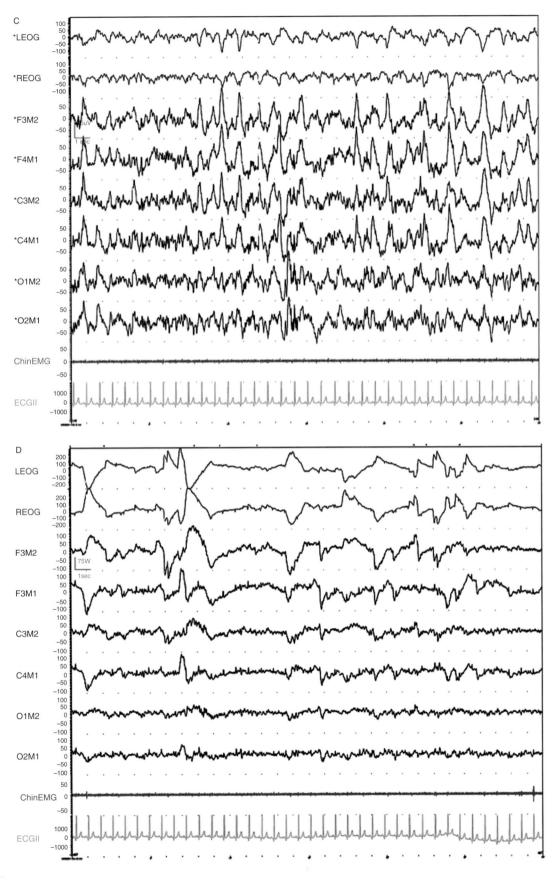

Epochs C–D.

Polysomnography findings in fibromyalgia

Neil Freedman

The 30 second PSG epoch shown is from a study in a patient with fibromyalgia.

Which one of the following statements is correct with reference to the finding identified by the brackets in the PSG epoch?

A. It is required for a diagnosis of fibromyalgia
B. It is both a sensitive and specific finding in this patient population
C. Its presence correlates with symptom severity
D. It may be reduced by treatment with sodium oxybate.

Answer on page 165.

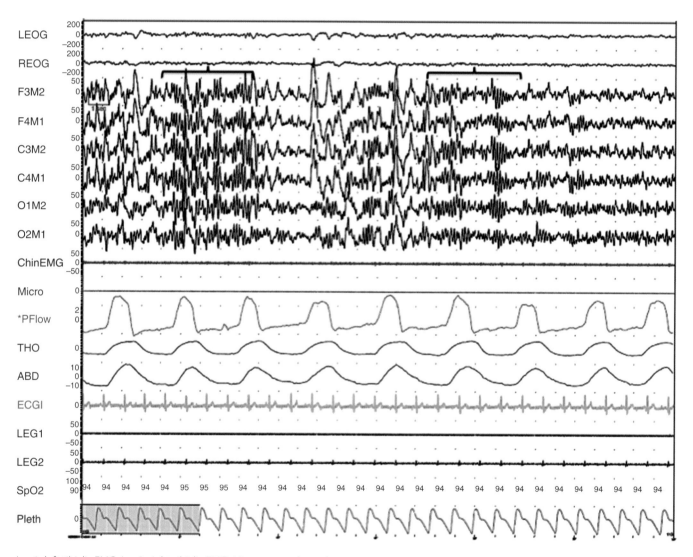

Leg1, left tibialis EMG; Leg2, right tibialis EMG; Micro, snore channel.

46 A 45-year-old man presents with newly diagnosed hypertension and symptoms of snoring

Neil Freedman

A 45-year-old man has symptoms of snoring and newly diagnosed hypertension. He denies daytime sleepiness, symptoms consistent with RLS, depression, neurologic complaints, abnormal behaviors during sleep, or alcohol use. His only medication is hydrochlorothiazide. His physical examination is notable for a BMI of 32 kg/m², and an oropharyngeal examination consistent with a Mallampati 3 classification.

He is sent for an overnight PSG, which does not demonstrate significant sleep-disordered breathing, abnormal EEG activity, or abnormal behaviors; however, it does demonstrate the following findings in this 30 second epoch.

Based on these PSG findings, what would be the best initial intervention?
A. Clonazepam at bedtime
B. Melatonin at bedtime
C. Venlafaxine at bedtime
D. No intervention at this time.

Answer on page 166.

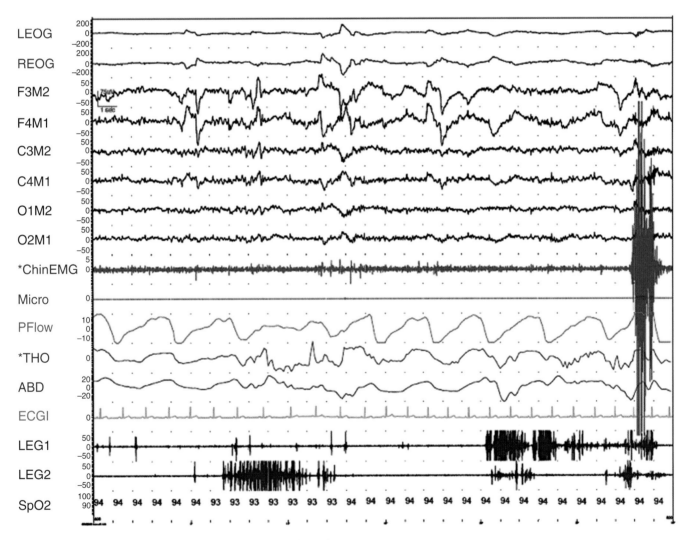

Leg1, left tibialis EMG; Leg2, right tibialis EMG; Micro, snore channel.

Case Studies in Polysomnography Interpretation, ed. Robert C. Basner. Published by Cambridge University Press. © Cambridge University Press 2012.

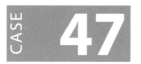
A 10-year-old child with central congenital hypoventilation syndrome

Fauziya Hassan and Ronald D. Chervin

The following 1 minute PSG tracing was recorded from a 10-year-old child with central congenital hypoventilation syndrome. The child recently received implanted phrenic nerve stimulators for diaphragmatic pacing. Hypoventilation had previously been managed by night-time mechanical ventilation through a tracheostomy. This study was performed with $ETCO_2$ monitoring. The tracheostomy was capped.

Based on this history and the interpretation of this PSG tracing, what is the most appropriate intervention to consider at this point in the study?
A. Uncap the tracheostomy
B. Lower the amplitude of the diaphragmatic pacers
C. Start bilevel PAP therapy via a mask
D. Wake the patient up
E. Change the patient's position.

Answer on page 166.

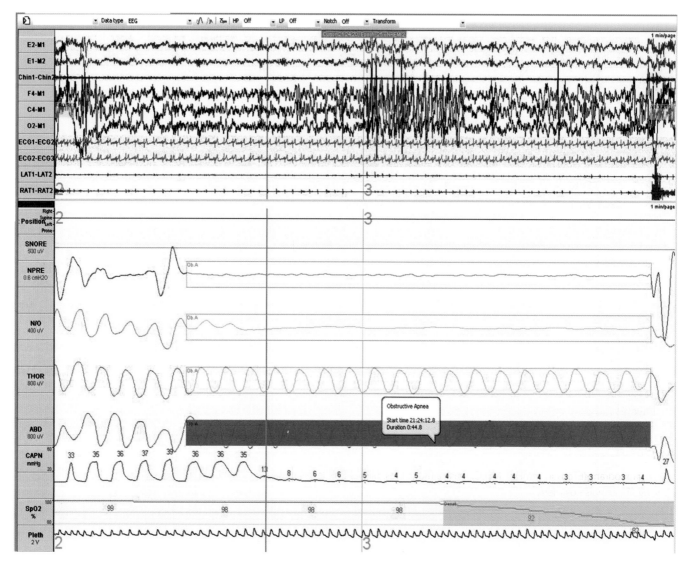

CAPN, capnogram ($ETCO_2$ tracing); N/O, oronasal thermocouple; NPRE, nasal pressure transducer; Position, body position; SpO_2 by finger pulse oximetry.

Case Studies in Polysomnography Interpretation, ed. Robert C. Basner. Published by Cambridge University Press. © Cambridge University Press 2012.

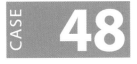
A 9-year-old child with asthma, skeletal dysplasia, restrictive lung disease, and obstructive sleep apnea

Fauziya Hassan and Ronald D. Chervin

A 9-year-old child with asthma and skeletal dysplasia with restrictive lung disease had a baseline PSG that showed OSA (AHI, 10.6/h; REM AHI, 60.7/h; O_2 desaturations to a nadir of 66%). The $ETCO_2$ values were in the 50 torr range during the study. During a subsequent PAP titration study, the following 1 minute PSG epoch was recorded.

Based on this information and interpretation of the PSG tracing, what is the most appropriate intervention to consider at this point in the titration?

A. Increase the pressure support on the bilevel PAP
B. Change the mask because leak is excessive
C. Change over to CPAP
D. Add a back-up rate in spontaneous timed mode or timed mode
E. Continue with the current setting.

Answer on page 167.

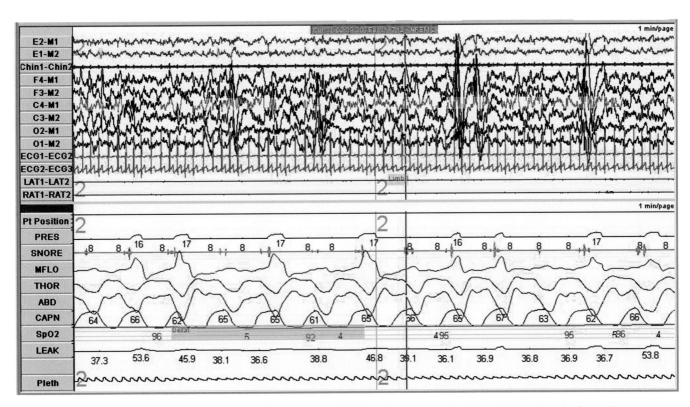

CAPN, capnogram ($ETCO_2$ in mmHg); MFLO, mask airflow; Pres, bilevel PAP levels that were administered; Pt position, body position; SpO_2 by finger pulse oximetry.

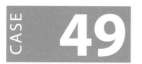

A 21-year-old man with a history of daytime sleepiness

Shelley Hershner

The following two epochs (each 60 seconds) are from the PSG of a 21-year-old man with a history of significant daytime sleepiness.

What is the most significant change from 1.5 hours after sleep onset to 4.5 hours after sleep onset, and what is the most likely etiology of this finding?

A. Increased fast frequency on the EEG; etiology is a medication effect, specifically the use of clonazepam

B. Enhanced volume and amplitude of slow waves; etiology is a medication effect, specifically the use of sodium oxybate

C. Increased low-voltage mixed frequency: REM sleep rebound from sleep deprivation

D. Increased spindle frequency; etiology is a medication effect, specifically the use of diazepam

E. Enhanced amount and amplitude of slow waves; etiology is a medication effect, specifically the use of zolpidem.

Answer on page 167.

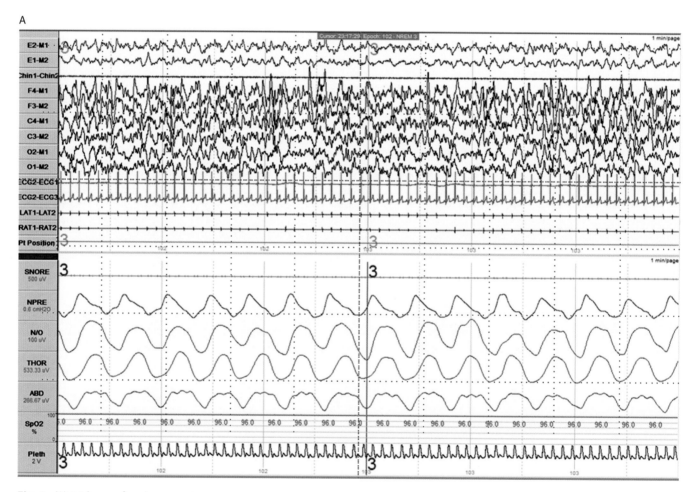

Fig. 1. (A) 1.5 hours after sleep onset.

B

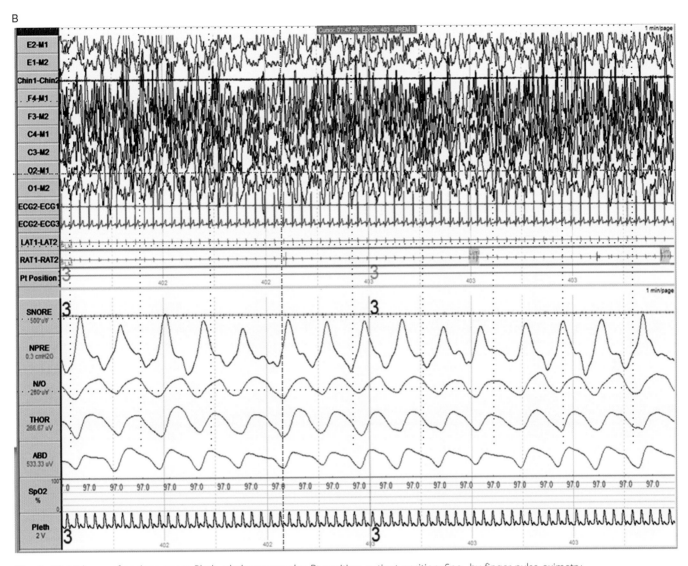

Fig. 1. (B) 4.5 hours after sleep onset. Pleth, plethysmography; Pt position, patient position; Spo₂ by finger pulse oximetry.

Shelley Hershner

A 58-year-old woman using a fentanyl patch and tramadol for chronic back pain presents with witnessed pauses in her breathing. A PSG is ordered. The following PSG tracing is a 60 second epoch from that PSG.

Which of the following statements is true about the PSG tracing displayed?

A. The tracing shows central sleep apnea; this is likely an opioid effect on respiration through the μ receptor

B. The PSG shows central sleep apnea, which is found in approximately 70% of patients taking opioids long term

C. The PSG shows central sleep apnea; opioids have been shown to increase both slow-wave sleep and REM sleep

D. The PSG shows central sleep apnea with Cheyne–Stokes breathing

E. The PSG shows central sleep apnea; opioid-induced respiratory depression decreases tidal volume more than respiratory rate.

Answer on page 168.

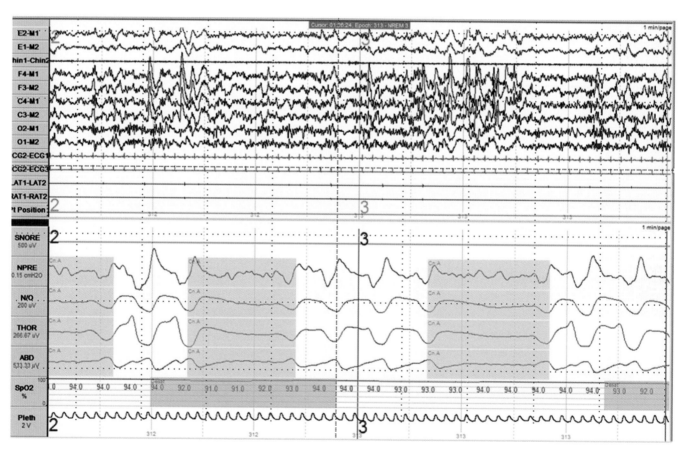

Pleth, plethysmography; Pt position, patient position; Spo₂ by finger pulse oximetry.

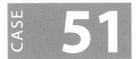
A 37-year-old woman with bipolar disorder and a recent head injury

David M. Hiestand and Satish C. Rao

The following two PSG tracings, the first a 30 second and the next a 10 second epoch, were recorded in a 37-year-old woman with witnessed snoring and poor sleep. She has a history of a head injury in the previous 6 weeks. She is currently taking lamotrigine for bipolar disorder. This epoch is representative of activity occurring several times early in the study.

What is the best interpretation of the activity displayed on these epochs?
A. Seizure activity
B. Periodic limb movements in sleep
C. Ocular artifact
D. Hypnagogic hypersynchrony
E. Frontal intermittent rhythmic delta activity.

Answer on page 169.

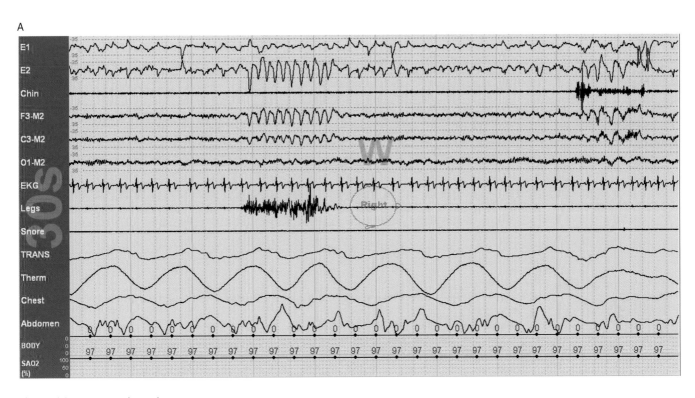

Fig. 1. (A) A 30 second epoch.

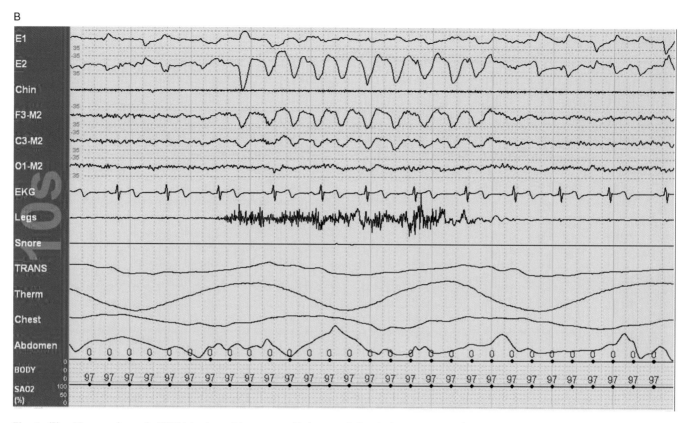

B

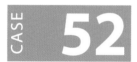

Fig. 1. (B) a 10 second epoch. BODY, body position sensor; Abdomen, abdominal respiratory inductance plethysmography; Legs, Leg EMG; Chest, thoracic respiratory inductance plethysmography; TRANS, nasal pressure transducer; SAO2, O₂ saturation by pulse oximetry.

CASE

52

A 12-year-old boy with a history of refractory seizures

David M. Hiestand and Kevin A. Thomas

The following PSG tracings were recorded in a 12-year-old boy with a history of refractory seizures. The patient has a BMI of 19 kg/m² and is known to snore. He is taking serotinergic antidepressant medication.

What is the best interpretation of the abnormal activity highlighted on these tracings?

A. Seizure activity
B. Vagal nerve stimulator artifact
C. REM sleep behavior disorder
D. Activity related to serotinergic antidepressants
E. Intermittent 60 Hz artifact.

Answer on page 170.

Case Studies in Polysomnography Interpretation, ed. Robert C. Basner. Published by Cambridge University Press. © Cambridge University Press 2012.

A

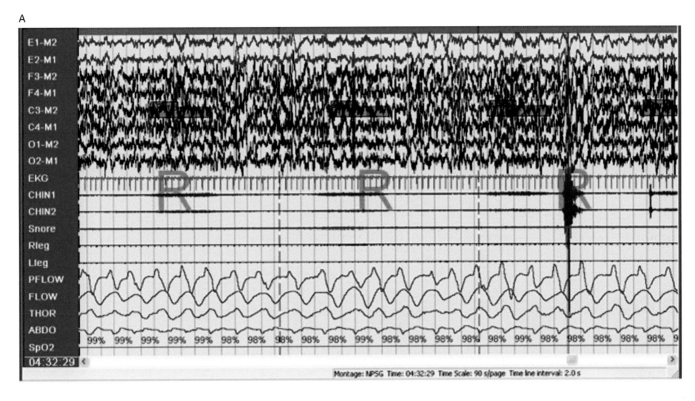

B

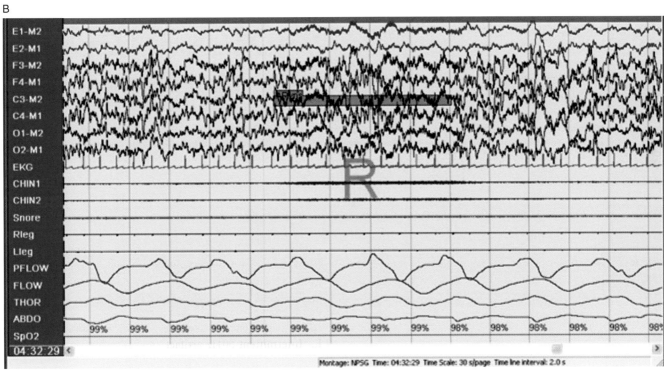

Fig. 1. (A) A 90 second epoch; (B) a 30 second epoch. Spo$_2$ by finger pulse oximetry.

An 8-year-old boy with snoring and poor sleep

David M. Hiestand and Kevin A. Thomas

The following epochs were recorded in an 8-year-old boy with snoring and poor sleep. His family reports that he has regular difficulty with sleep onset associated with marked physical activity. The following two PSG epochs are representative of activity occurring in each of the awake periods (Fig. 1A and B) and is demonstrated on the hypnogram (Fig. 1C); the activity usually continues during the study 1–2 minutes at a time.

What is the best interpretation of the activity displayed on these PSG epochs?

A. Seizure
B. Hypnagogic jerks
C. Sweat artifact
D. Body rocking
E. Night terrors.

Answer on page 170.

A

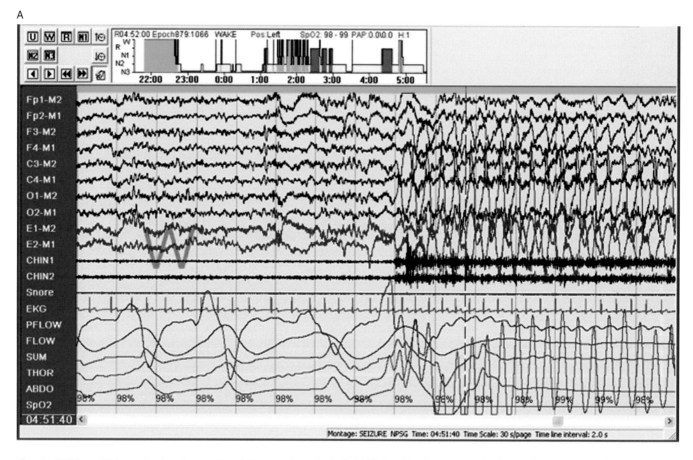

Fig. 1. (A,B) Two PSG epochs showing activity during awake periods. Fp1-M2, Fp2-M1, frontoparietal referential EEG; Spo₂ by finger pulse oximetry.

B

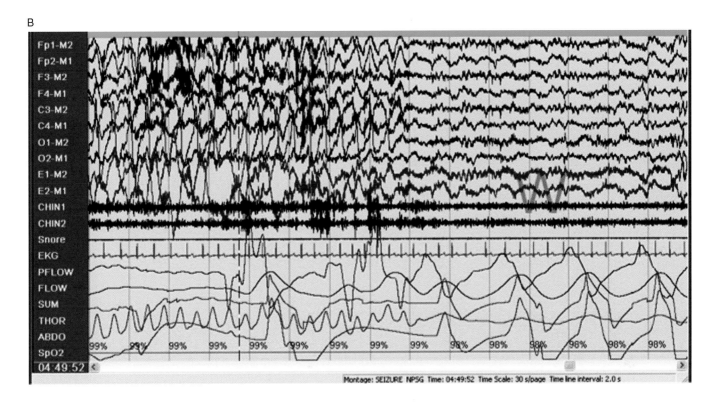

C

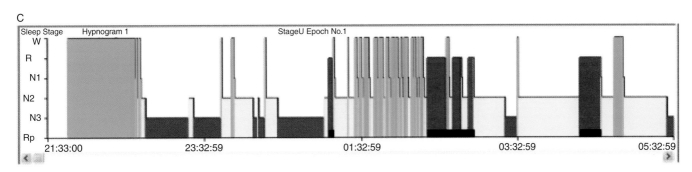

Fig. 1. (C) hypnogram.

54 A 30-week premature infant with snoring and poor sleep at 17 months of age

David M. Hiestand and Kevin A. Thomas

The following epoch was recorded in a 17-month-old boy with snoring and poor sleep. He was born prematurely at 30 weeks of gestation. His family reports regular difficulty with sleep onset as well as frequent awakenings. The following 90 second PSG epoch is representative of activity occurring throughout sleep, but most prominent in REM periods.

What is the best interpretation of the activity displayed on this epoch?

A. Respiratory effort-related arousals
B. Obstructive apneas
C. Cheyne–Stokes breathing
D. Mixed apneas
E. Periodic breathing.

Answer on page 171.

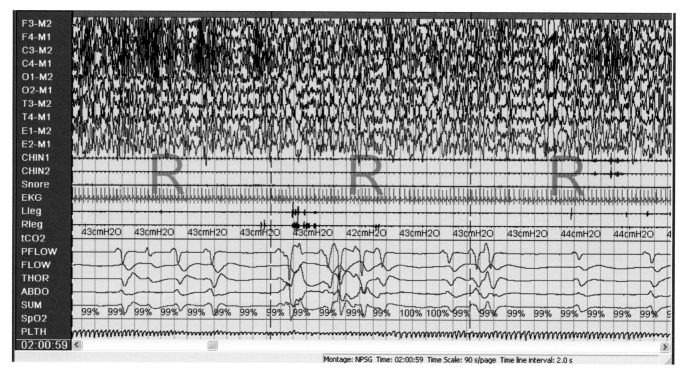

PFLOW, pressure transducer signal; FLOW, oronasal thermistor; T3-M2, T4-M1, temporal referential EEG; tCO2, transcutaneous CO_2; PLTH, plethysmography; Spo2 by finger pulse oximetry.

Case Studies in Polysomnography Interpretation, ed. Robert C. Basner. Published by Cambridge University Press. © Cambridge University Press 2012.

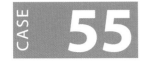

A 75-year-old man with a history of excessive daytime sleepiness and generalized body "weakness" with excitement, surprise, and anger

Mithri Junna and Timothy I. Morgenthaler

Shown below are a 30 second epoch and hypnogram from a PSG completed in a 75-year-old man with a history of consistent excessive daytime sleepiness for 60 years, generalized body "weakness" with excitement, surprise, and anger for 50 years, and dream-enactment behavior for 5 years. He has no other abnormal medical history.

Which of the following is the most likely diagnosis using this history and interpretation of the tracings?
A. Narcolepsy
B. Idiopathic hypersomnia with long sleep time
C. Idiopathic hypersomnia without long sleep time
D. Kleine–Levin syndrome.

Answer on page 171.

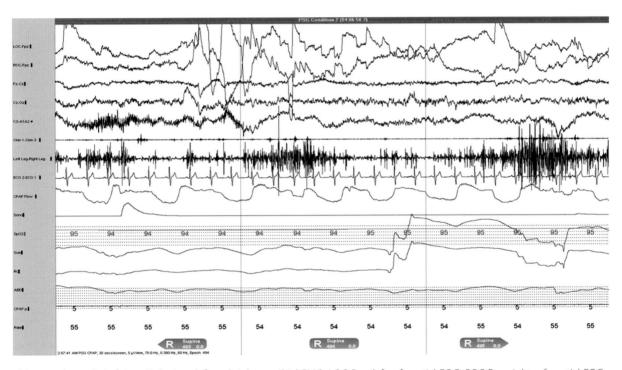

Fig. 1. 30 second epoch. Left Leg-Right Leg, left and right pretibial EMG; LOC-Fpz, left referential EOG; ROC-Fpz, right referential EOG; RC, thoracic respiratory effort; Rate, heart rate.

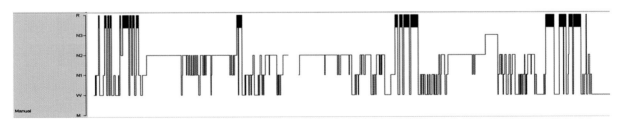

Fig. 2. Hypnogram. R, REM sleep; N1, NREM stage 1; N2, NREM stage 2; N3, NREM stage 3; W, awake.

An 18-year-old woman with a 2 year history of being a "late sleeper"

Mithri Junna and Timothy I. Morgenthaler

Shown below is a 2 week actigraphy study from an 18-year-old woman with a history of being a "late sleeper" over 2 years. During the school week, she often goes to bed at midnight and awakens feeling unrefreshed at 6:30 a.m., supplementing this with a 30 minute nap in the evenings. During the weekends, she often goes to bed at 2:00 a.m. and awakens feeling refreshed at 11 a.m.

Based on this history and the interpretation of the actigraphy shown, which of the following is the most likely diagnosis?
A. Delayed sleep phase disorder
B. Advanced sleep phase disorder
C. Irregular sleep–wake circadian rhythm sleep disorder
D. Free-running or non-entrained circadian rhythm disorder.

Answer on page 172.

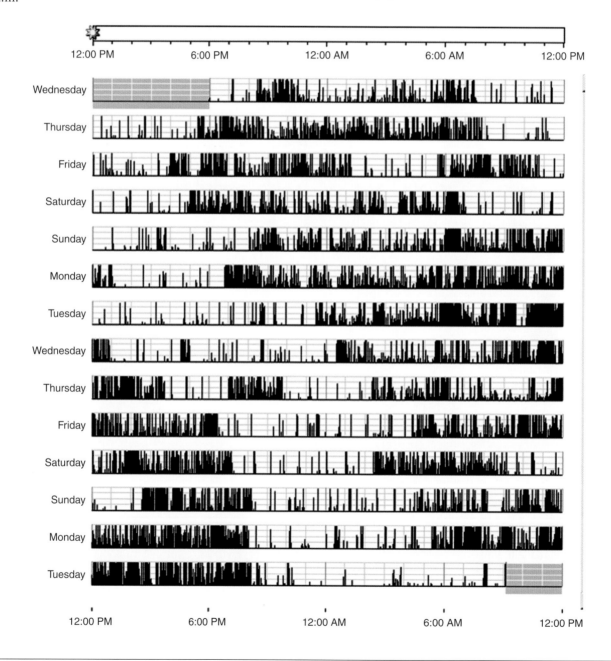

Case Studies in Polysomnography Interpretation, ed. Robert C. Basner. Published by Cambridge University Press. © Cambridge University Press 2012.

An otherwise healthy 9-year-old boy who falls asleep in school

Kristen Kelly-Pieper and Carin Lamm

An otherwise healthy 9-year-old boy is evaluated for falling asleep in school. He developed weakness and hypersomnia 1 year earlier following a febrile viral illness. The episodes of weakness are described as eyelid droopiness when very tired or laughing. Work-up for myasthenia gravis was negative. He denies snoring, vivid dreams, and unusual limb movements. He is currently not taking any medications.

Sleep logs were obtained for 2 weeks leading up to the nocturnal PSG with MSLT. The sleep logs showed a typical nocturnal sleep period from 9:30 p.m. to 7:00 a.m. with several brief awakenings during the night. Multiple short daytime naps were present. Overnight PSG (total sleep time > 7 hours) was performed, which demonstrated fragmented sleep but no evidence of sleep-disordered breathing or

abnormal leg movements. A five nap MSLT was performed the following morning, which resulted in sleep in all naps with a mean sleep latency of 2 minutes. The following tracing (30 seconds) from his MSLT is representative of epochs that were present in three out of five nap opportunities.

What is the most accurate ICSD diagnosis based on the interpretation of the PSG tracing shown and this history?

A. Narcolepsy without cataplexy
B. Idiopathic hypersomnia without long sleep time
C. Recurrent hypersomnia (Kleine–Levin syndrome)
D. Delayed sleep phase disorder
E. Behaviorally induced insufficient sleep syndrome.

Answer on page 172.

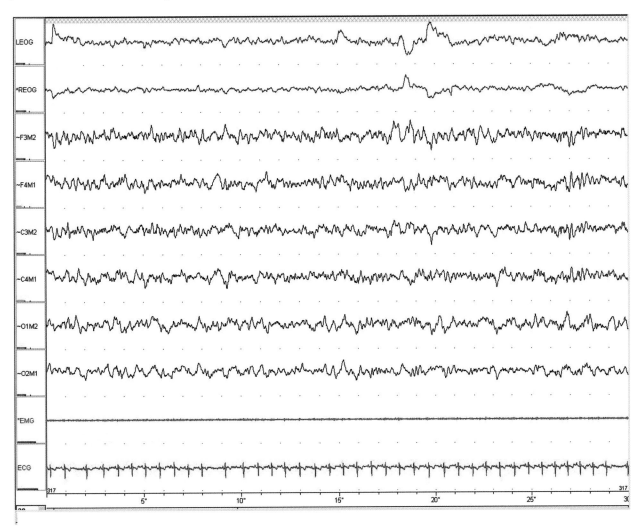

Case Studies in Polysomnography Interpretation, ed. Robert C. Basner. Published by Cambridge University Press. © Cambridge University Press 2012.

A 35-year-old woman who is 6 months pregnant and has a history of snoring with pauses in breathing

Douglas Kirsch

A 35-year-old woman comes to the sleep center for an evaluation for OSA. Her husband reports that she has been a long time snorer but that, over the last few months, she has had notably louder snoring as well as new pauses in her breathing during the night. Her snoring used to be positional, but now both snoring and pauses appear not to be affected by position. These symptoms have correlated with weight gain as part of her pregnancy, in which she is now in the sixth month. She is unaware of any of the symptoms, other than when her husband wakes her up telling her to start breathing. She denies significant excessive daytime sleepiness but notes that she has been more "tired" during her pregnancy.

Her examination demonstrates normal vital signs. Her BMI is elevated at 32. She has a 41.2 cm (16.5 inch) circumference neck. She has a Mallampati class 4 airway, with a high arched hard palate and long soft palate. She has mild retrognathia. Her sleep study demonstrates the following images: Fig. 1A

is a 30 second epoch during stage W (biocals) and Fig. 1B is a 30 second epoch during stage R sleep.

1. What is the identifiable artifact on both these PSG tracings?
A. 60 Hz artifact
B. ECG artifact
C. EOG artifact
D. M1 artifact
E. Sweat sway artifact.

2. How are REMs defined?
A. Regular and sinusoidal appearance
B. A slow phase followed by a rapid phase
C. An initial movement usually lasting < 500 milliseconds
D. Disconjugate eye movements
E. Occurrence solely during stage R sleep.

Answer on page 173.

A

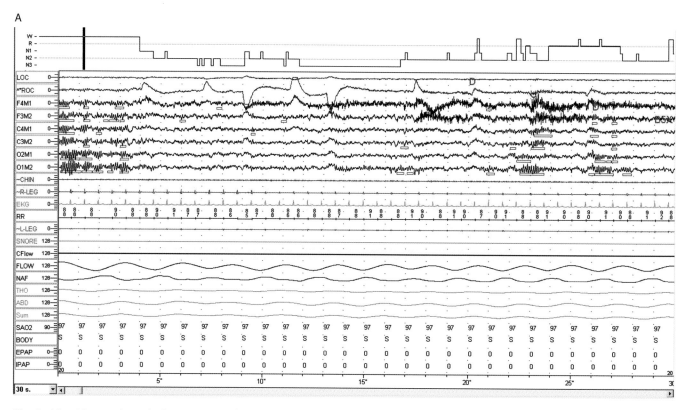

Fig. 1. (A) a 30 second epoch during stage W (biocals).

Case Studies in Polysomnography Interpretation, ed. Robert C. Basner. Published by Cambridge University Press. © Cambridge University Press 2012.

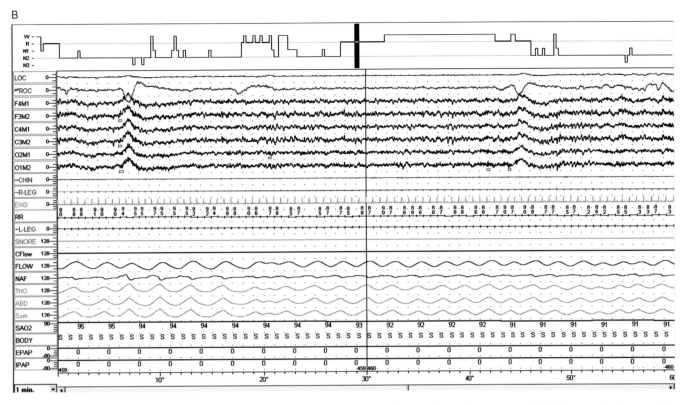

Fig. 1. (B) a 30 second epoch during stage R sleep. Flow, oronasal thermistor; RR, pulse rate from pulse oximeter; SAO2, O₂ saturation by ear pulse oximetry.

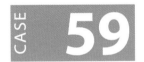

CASE 59

A 22-year-old graduate student with daytime tiredness

Douglas Kirsch

A 22-year-old graduate student presents to the sleep center with complaints of daytime tiredness. He has been having problems with alertness during the daytime for the last few years, increasing to the point where he is napping daily. He has difficulty driving for longer than 15 minutes because of drowsiness. He denies snoring or gasping episodes, although he has no bed partner to currently confirm the absence of these symptoms. He denies hypnagogic hallucinations and cataplexy, but does note occasional sleep paralysis. He denies RLS symptoms.

His overnight PSG demonstrates a sleep efficiency of 93% with 8 hours of recording time, and no sleep-disordered breathing. A histogram of his daytime mean sleep latency test is shown in Fig. 1 and a representative 30 second PSG epoch occurring at minute 7 of the first nap of his MSLT in Fig. 2.

Which one of the following statements is correct regarding the interpretation of these findings in this setting?

A. These findings rule out the diagnosis of narcolepsy without cataplexy

B. These data are invalid to assess for narcolepsy as only four naps were completed

C. These data are compatible with narcolepsy without cataplexy

D. These findings are invalid to assess for narcolepsy based on his previous night's sleep results.

Answer on page 173.

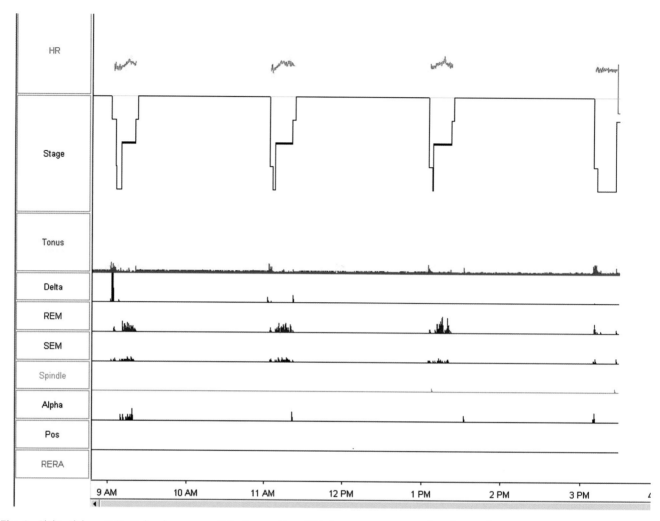

Fig. 1. Alpha, alpha activity; Delta, slow wave activity; Pos, position; SEM, slow eye movements; Spindle, spindle activity; Stage, sleep stage; Tonus, chin EMG.

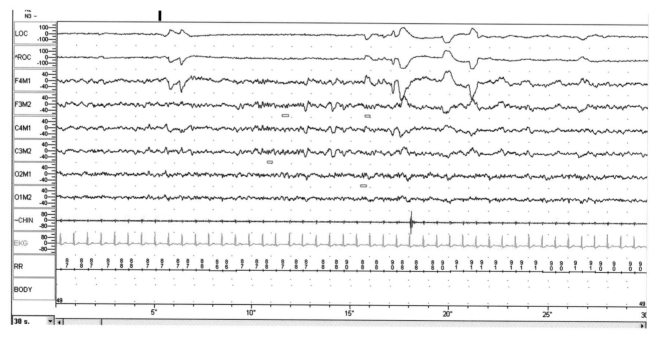

Fig. 2. RR, pulse rate from pulse oximeter.

Interpretation of traces from polysomnography

Brian B. Koo and Kingman Strohl

A patient has the following hypnogram from a PSG (Fig. 1) and a representative 30 second epoch from the PSG (Fig. 2).

Which of the following best describes this patient, based on interpretation of these tracings?

A. A 78-year-old man with congestive heart failure
B. A 54-year-old man with end-stage amyotrophic lateral sclerosis

C. A 33-year-old woman with obesity
D. A 7-year-old girl with seizures
E. A 35-year-old man with obesity.

Answer on page 174.

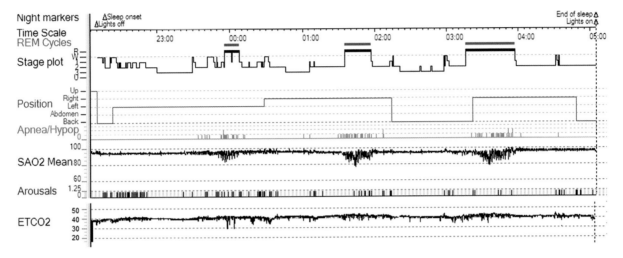

Fig. 1. Hypnogram.

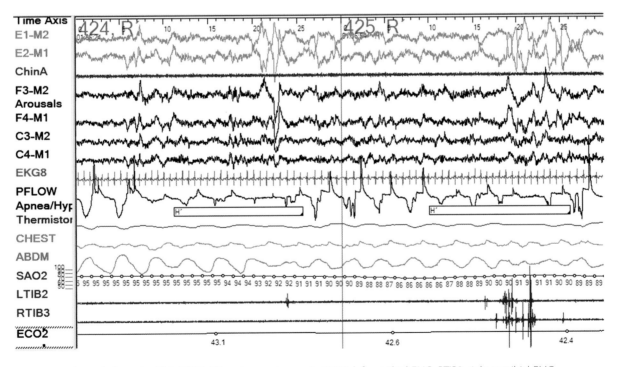

Fig. 2. A 30 second epoch from the PSG. ECO2, ETco$_2$ by nasal cannula; LTIB2, left pretibial EMG; RTIB3, right pretibial EMG.

Case Studies in Polysomnography Interpretation, ed. Robert C. Basner. Published by Cambridge University Press. © Cambridge University Press 2012.

An adult being assessed for obstructive sleep apnea

Brian B. Koo and Kingman Strohl

An adult being assessed for OSA had the 60 second PSG epoch shown below.

Which of the following is the best interpretation of the breathing marked with an asterisk?

A. Hypopnea
B. Central apnea
C. Normal breathing
D. Cheyne–Stokes breathing.

Answer on page 174.

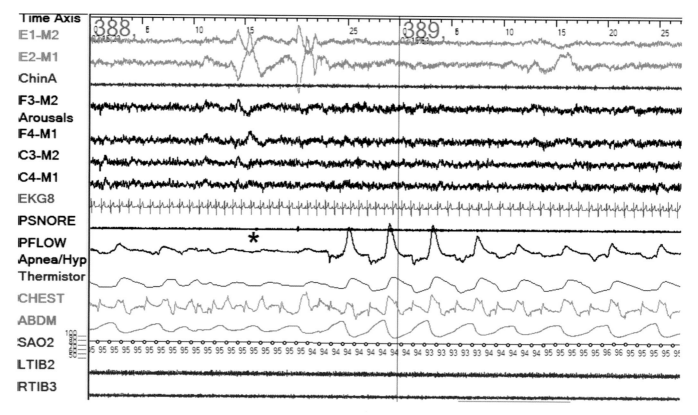

LTIB2, left pretibialis EMG; RTIB3, right pretibialis EMG.

Case Studies in Polysomnography Interpretation, ed. Robert C. Basner. Published by Cambridge University Press. © Cambridge University Press 2012.

A 22-year-old woman with a 2 year history of motor activity during sleep that is increasing in frequency

Raman Malhotra and Shalini Paruthi

A 22-year-old woman has a 2 year history of motor activity during sleep, which has been increasing in frequency over the last several months. She is amnestic of the events but is told she converses with others or sometimes moves items around the room during sleep.

During overnight attended PSG, the patient had a typical spell of sitting up in bed and speaking nonsense. Figure 1 is a 30 second epoch from the sleep study depicting the onset of the event.

1. Given the above history and PSG interpretation, what is the most likely diagnosis?

A. Complex partial seizures
B. REM sleep behavior disorder
C. NREM sleep parasomnia
D. Sleep-related dissociative disorder
E. Nightmare disorder.

A further 30 second PSG fragment is shown in Fig. 2.

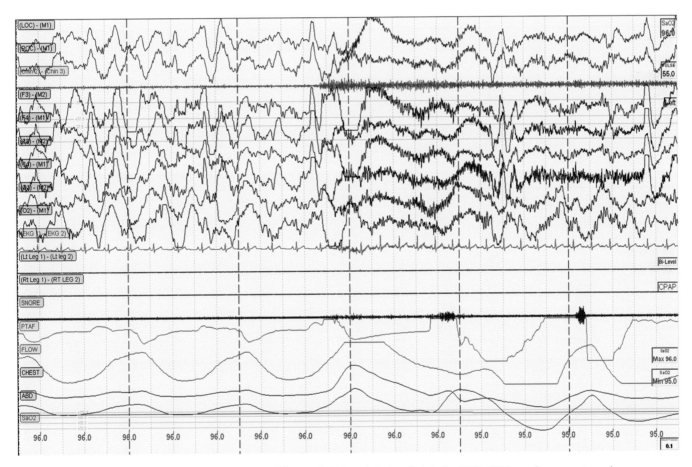

Fig. 1. Flow, oronasal thermistor; Lt Leg 1–Lt Leg 2, left leg EMG; Rt Leg 1–Rt Leg 2, right leg EMG; PTAF, nasal pressure transducer.

Case Studies in Polysomnography Interpretation, ed. Robert C. Basner. Published by Cambridge University Press. © Cambridge University Press 2012.

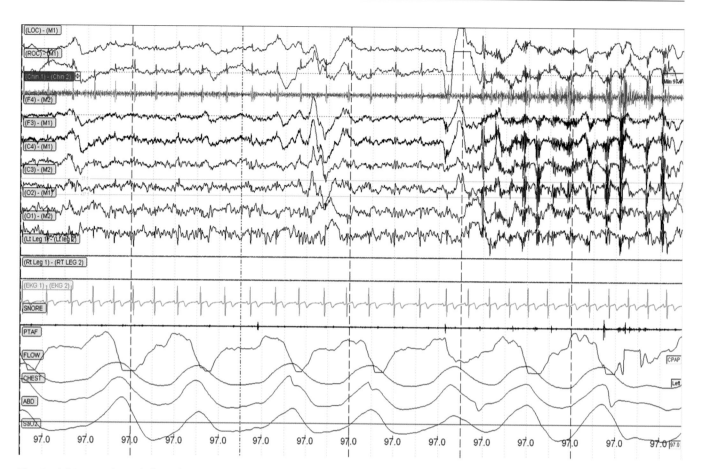

Fig. 2. A 30 second epoch from the same PSG. Flow, oronasal thermistor; Lt Leg 1–Lt Leg 2, left leg EMG; Rt Leg 1–Rt Leg 2, right leg EMG.

2. What finding is suggested on this 30 second PSG fragment?

A. REM sleep without muscle atonia
B. Sleep-related bruxism
C. A 60 Hz artifact
D. Electrode popping
E. Epileptiform activity.

Answer on page 175.

63 A 43-year-old woman with a 2 year history of unusual motor activity during sleep

Raman Malhotra and Shalini Paruthi

A 43-year-old woman presents with a 2 year history of unusual motor activity reported by her spouse. The spouse reports that she yells, screams, kicks, and sometimes punches during sleep. Her overnight PSG showed an AHI of 5.8/h and minimum SpO_2 of 88%. Her REM sleep AHI was 21.3/h. She had decreased sleep efficiency of 68%, with decreased REM sleep percentage of 8% of total sleep time. The following is a 1 minute tracing from her PSG.

Given the history and the interpretation of the PSG tracing, what is the most likely diagnosis?

A. Sleep-walking
B. Idiopathic RBD
C. Sleep-related epilepsy
D. Pseudo-REM sleep behavior caused by OSA
E. Non-epileptic spell (pseudoseizure).

Answer on page 176.

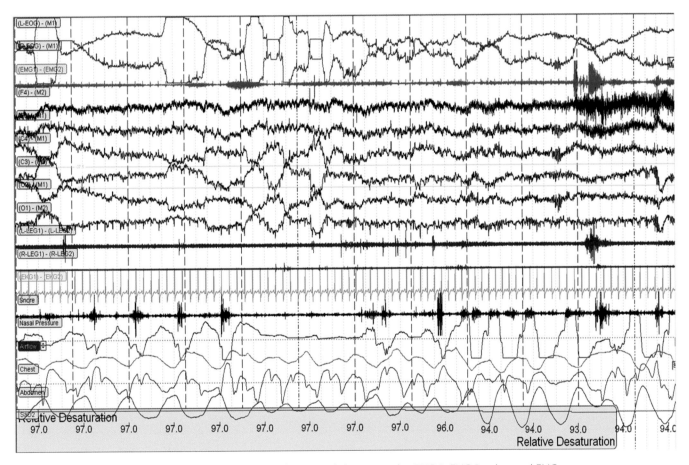

Airflow, oronasal thermistor; Chest, thoracic respiratory inductance plethysmography; EMG 1–EMG 2, submental EMG.

A 28-year-old man with spells of nonsensical speech and clumsy motor activity at night

Raman Malhotra and Shalini Paruthi

A 28-year-old man reports having spells at night that have occurred over the previous year. His bed partner describes nonsensical speech and clumsy motor activity. The patient is amnestic of the events. A nocturnal PSG showed an AHI of 1.8/h, minimum SpO_2 of 92%, and normal sleep architecture with sleep efficiency of 92%. No typical spells were recorded; however, the patient had an increased amount of spontaneous arousals, at 24 cortical arousals per hour. A representative tracing of his typical arousals are shown below in this 30 second PSG epoch.

Based upon the above history and interpretation of the PSG tracing, what are these spells most consistent with?

A. REM sleep behavior disorder
B. Sleep-related panic attacks
C. Complex partial seizures
D. Confusional arousal
E. Obstructive sleep apnea.

Answer on page 176.

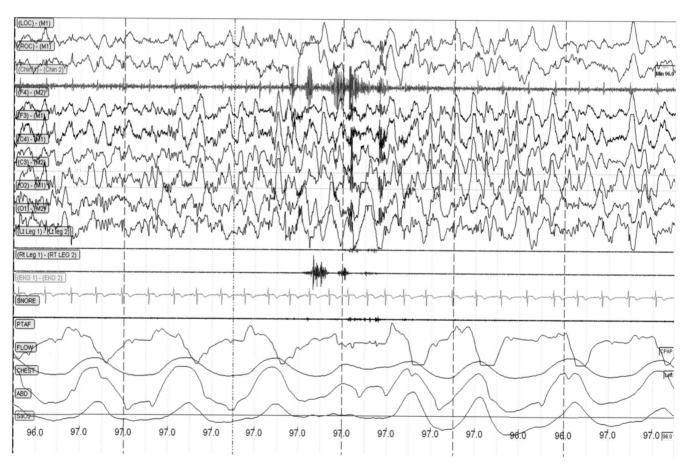

FLOW, oronasal thermistor; Lt Leg 1–Lt Leg 2, left leg EMG; Rt Leg 1–Rt Leg 2, right leg EMG.

A 5-year-old child who frequently shakes and cries in her sleep

Raman Malhotra and Shalini Paruthi

A 5-year-old child is noted to shake at night and cry in her sleep frequently, up to four times a night, approximately six nights per week. A 10 second epoch from the nocturnal PSG obtained in this child is shown.

What is the most likely diagnosis given the above history and interpretation of the PSG tracing shown?
A. Epilepsy
B. REM sleep behavior disorder
C. Hypnagogic foot tremor
D. Fragmentary myoclonus.

Answer on page 177.

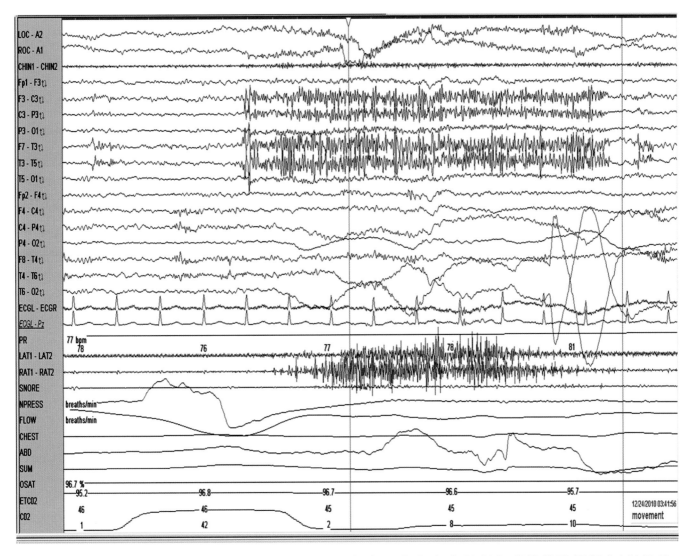

CO2, capnography signal; PR, heart rate; extended EEG montage covers leads Fp1-F3, F3-C3, C3-P3, P3-O1, F7-T3, T3-T5, T5-O1, Fp2-F4, F4-C4, C4-P4, P4-O2, F8-T4, T4-T6, T6-O2.

Case Studies in Polysomnography Interpretation, ed. Robert C. Basner. Published by Cambridge University Press. © Cambridge University Press 2012.

A 45-year-old man with a history of gastroesophageal reflux disease taking methadone who has snoring, witnessed apnea, and excessive daytime sleepiness

Meghna P. Mansukhani and Timothy I. Morgenthaler

A 45-year-old man with a medical history of significant gastro-esophageal reflux disease is taking oral methadone at a dosage of 30 mg three times a day. He has been taking this for the last 2 years for chronic back pain. He presents now with a history of snoring, witnessed apneas, and excessive daytime sleepiness. His BMI is 35 kg/m² and his oropharynx appears crowded on examination, with a Friedman class III palatal position.

He undergoes PSG and a representative tracing (approximately 5 minutes) from his PSG is shown below.

What is the most accurate interpretation of the respiratory abnormality in this tracing?

A. Cheyne–Stokes breathing
B. Cluster breathing
C. Biot's breathing
D. Apneustic breathing
E. Primary central sleep apnea.

Answer on page 177.

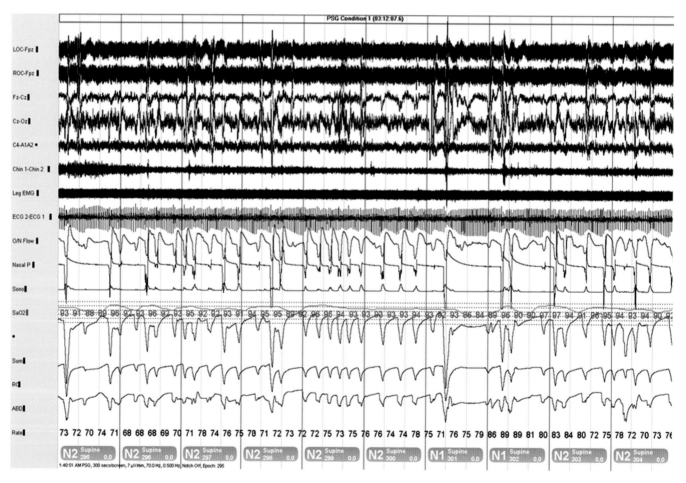

Leg EMG, pretibial EMG; LOC-Fpz, left referential EOG; ROC-Fpz, right referential EOG; O/N flow, oronasal airflow; Rate, heart rate; RC, thoracic respiratory effort.

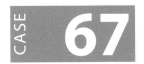
A 49-year-old man with possible sleep apnea

Jean K. Matheson

The following 60 second PSG epoch was recorded in a 49-year-old man who was being assessed for potential sleep apnea. A brief episode of sudden loud yelling and shouting was observed by the technician (see notation on PSG), soon followed by the patient awakening to make a trip to the bathroom.

Based on this history and interpretation of the PSG tracing, what is the most likely diagnosis for this behavior?

A. REM sleep behavior disorder
B. Confusional arousal
C. Sleep terror
D. Panic attack.

Answer on page 178.

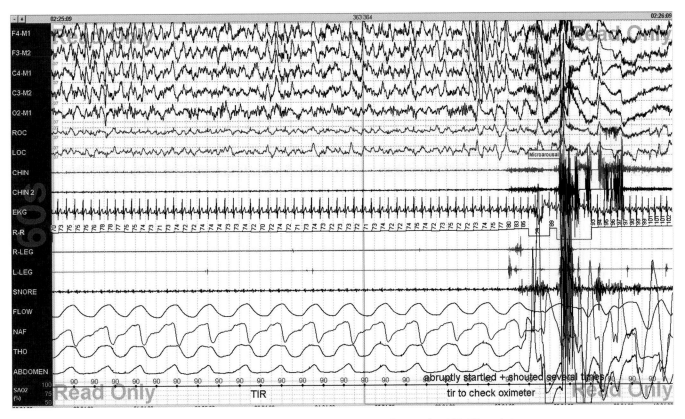

Flow, oronasal thermistor; NAF, nasal pressure transducer air flow; R-R, heart rate from pulse ECG; TIR, tech in room.

Case Studies in Polysomnography Interpretation, ed. Robert C. Basner. Published by Cambridge University Press. © Cambridge University Press 2012.

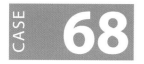
A 25-year-old morbidly obese man with loud snoring and excessive daytime sleepiness

Jean K. Matheson

The 60 second PSG epoch below was recorded in a 25-year-old morbidly obese man who complained of loud snoring and excessive daytime sleepiness.

How are these ECG abnormalities best reported?

A. The ECG cannot be interpreted because of artifact secondary to an apnea and an arousal

B. Paroxysmal atrial tachycardia secondary to an arousal

C. Bradycardia secondary to an obstructive apnea followed by ECG artifact

D. Bradycardia secondary to an obstructive apnea followed by atrial fibrillation.

Answer on page 179.

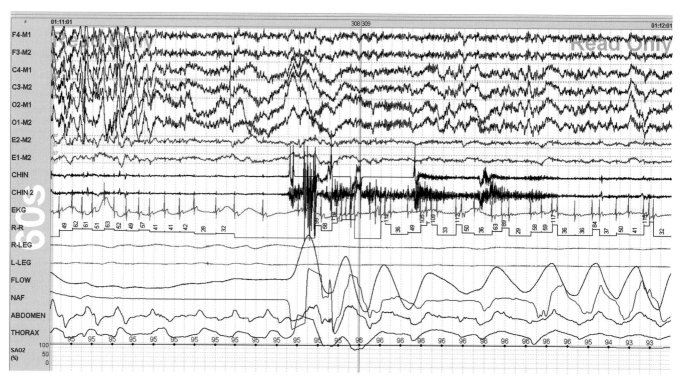

Abdomen, abdominal respiratory piezoelectric bands; Flow, oronasal thermistor; R-R, heart rate from pulse oximetry; THORAX, thoracic respiratory piezoelectric bands; SAO2, Spo$_2$ by finger pulse oximetry.

A 55-year-old man with snoring and excessive daytime sleepiness

Gökhan M. Mutlu and Lisa Wolfe

A 55-year-old man was referred for PSG because of complaints of snoring and excessive daytime sleepiness. During the recording, a standard AASM montage was utilized including six EEG leads, a oronasal thermistor, nasal pressure transducer, and respiratory inductance plethysmography. Two epochs from NREM sleep are displayed: Fig. 1A is the first epoch of 30 seconds; Fig. 1B, the second epoch, is displayed at a faster speed and is 5 seconds long.

What is the best interpretation for the cause of the artifact seen in the chest lead?

A. A 60 Hz artifact from the head box

B. Snoring artifact

C. Pulse artifact

D. Electrical artifact from the respiratory inductance plethysmography module.

Answer on page 179.

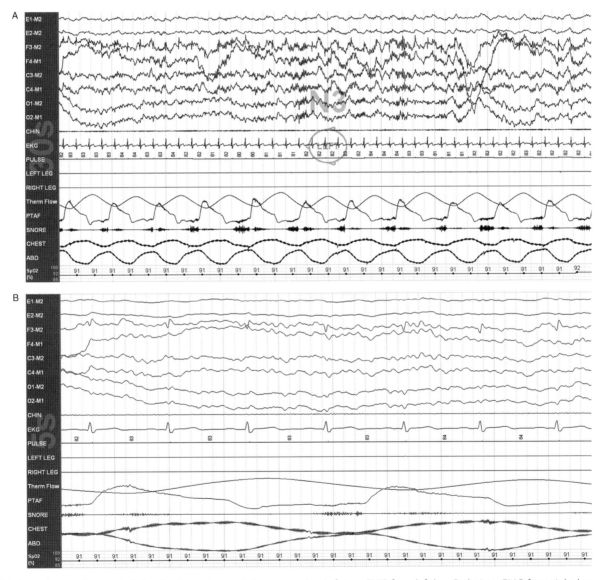

Chest/Abd, respiratory chest and abdominal inductance plethysmography; Left Leg, EMG from left leg; Right Leg, EMG from right leg.

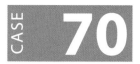
A 61-year-old woman with loud snoring and daytime sleepiness

Gökhan M. Mutlu and Lisa Wolfe

A 61-year-old woman with complaints of loud snoring and daytime sleepiness was referred for PSG. She also had complaints of motor restlessness but denied any issues with sleep disruption from this feeling. Below is a 30 second epoch of NREM sleep recorded during her diagnostic study.

What is the best interpretation of the findings seen in the right leg EMG?

A. A 60 Hz artifact
B. Hypnic foot tremor
C. Periodic limb movements
D. Restless legs syndrome.

Answer on page 180.

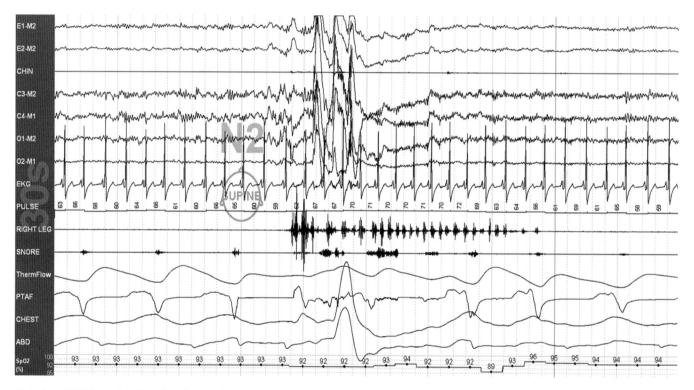

Right Leg, EMG from right leg; Spo₂ from pulse oximetry.

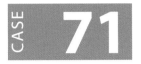

CASE 71

A 50-year-old woman with a complaint of daytime sleepiness

Gökhan M. Mutlu and Lisa Wolfe

The PSG epochs below were recorded from a 50-year-old woman with a complaint of daytime sleepiness. Her medications included citalopram, benztropine, lorazepam, cyclobenzaprine, valsartan, amlodipine, diphenhydramine, temazepam, budesonide plus formoterol, and albuterol. The first epoch below (A) is from the first REM period of the study (epoch 838). The second epoch (B) is a 1 minute recording during representative NREM sleep.

Which medication is most likely to explain the findings in the PSG epoch and the history?

A. Valsartan-related cough, hypoxemia, and snoring
B. Albuterol-related tachycardia, arousals, and upper airway resistance
C. Citalopram-related delay in REM onset, high chin EMG tone, and NREM PLMs
D. Lorazepam-related giant spindles in REM sleep, alpha intrusion in NREM, and PLMs.

Answer on page 180.

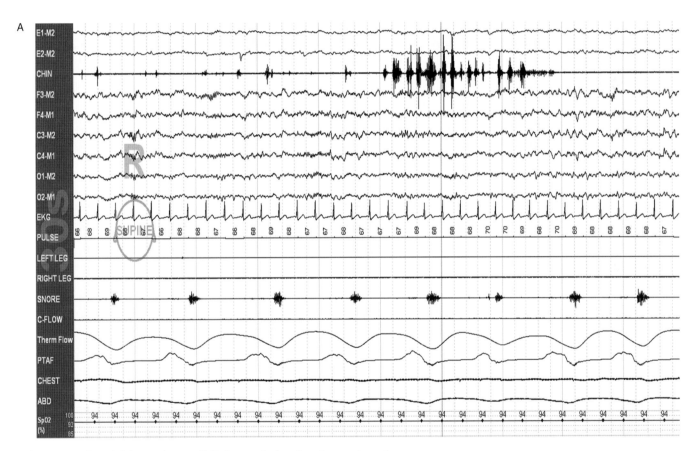

Left Leg, EMG from left leg; Right Leg, EMG from right leg; Spo₂ from pulse oximetry.

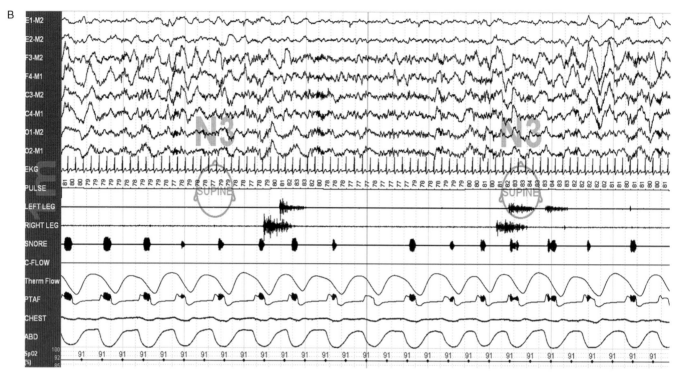

(cont.)

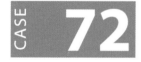

A 50-year-old obese man with a history of left ventricular failure and witnessed apnea

Gökhan M. Mutlu and Lisa Wolfe

A 50-year-old obese man (BMI of 39 kg/m^2) with history of left ventricular failure is referred for PSG because of the occurrence of witnessed apnea. He was found to have severe OSA and a CPAP titration was initiated. Because of pressure intolerance, he was switched to bilevel PAP therapy. Below is a 2 minute epoch of REM sleep during the bilevel PAP titration (IPAP/EPAP, 17/10 cmH$_2$O).

Which statement related to the finding shown by the arrow is correct?
A. Supplementation with nocturnal O_2 or CO_2 would directly resolve this finding
B. This finding is caused by increased respiratory efforts
C. Increasing IPAP will resolve this respiratory event
D. Daytime $Paco_2$ is likely low in this patient.

Answer on page 181.

Case Studies in Polysomnography Interpretation, ed. Robert C. Basner. Published by Cambridge University Press. © Cambridge University Press 2012.

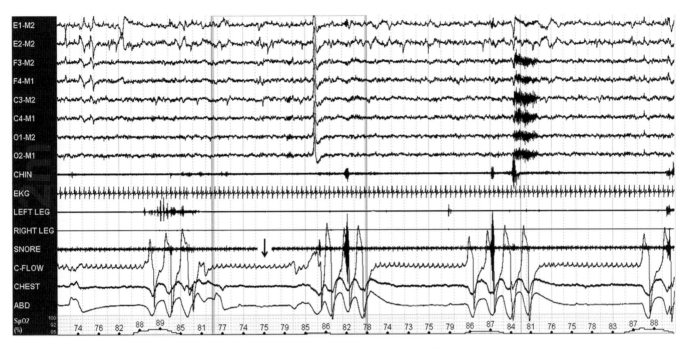

C-Flow, nasal thermistor; Left Leg, EMG from left leg; Right Leg, EMG from right leg; Spo₂ from pulse oximetry.

CASE 73

A 34-year-old man with snoring and excessive sleepiness

Gökhan M. Mutlu and Lisa Wolfe

A 34-year-old man with no significant cardiac or respiratory past medical history underwent PSG for evaluation of snoring and excessive sleepiness. A 2 minute epoch (A) and a 30 second epoch (B) from the PSG are shown.

Which of the following statements regarding the respiratory findings displayed is correct?

A. These are obstructive hypopneas
B. A $\geq$ 4% desaturation in O_2 saturation is required for the diagnosis of these events
C. The presence of an arousal is required for the diagnosis of these events
D. These are not a cause of hypersomnia.

Answer on page 181.

Case Studies in Polysomnography Interpretation, ed. Robert C. Basner. Published by Cambridge University Press. © Cambridge University Press 2012.

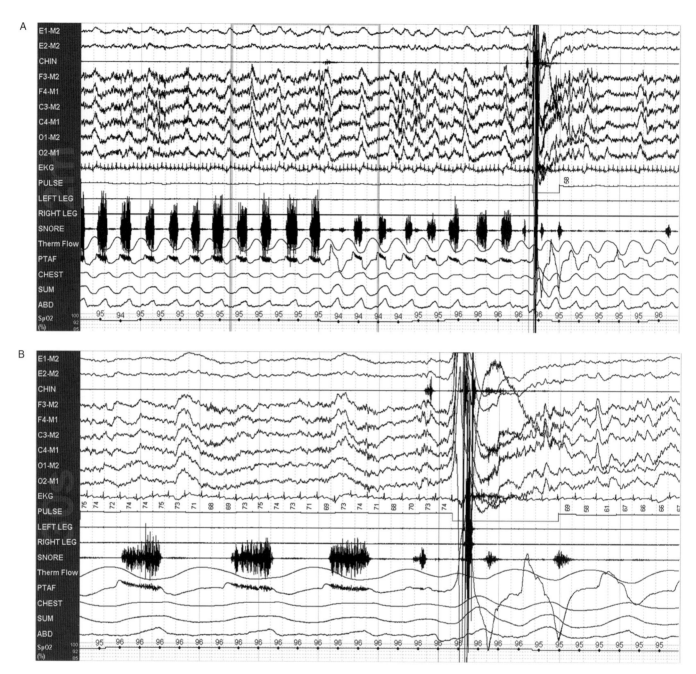

Left Leg, EMG from left leg; Right Leg, EMG from right leg; Spo₂ from pulse oximetry.

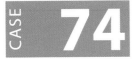
A 55-year-old man with a T11 spinal cord injury and paraplegia in association with metastatic disease, complaining of daytime sleepiness

Gökhan M. Mutlu and Lisa Wolfe

A 55-year-old man with a T11 spinal cord injury and paraplegia in association with metastatic disease is referred for a PSG because of complaints of daytime sleepiness. The study showed severe sleep apnea, and after 2 hours of recording, a CPAP titration was initiated. A 2 minute epoch of NREM sleep recorded during the CPAP titration is shown.

Which statement regarding the finding in the right leg lead is correct?
A. This finding represents snore artifact
B. These events are PLMs
C. Leg leads do not need to be monitored during PSG in patients with known spinal cord injury
D. This finding results from basal ganglia related abnormalities.

Answer on page 182.

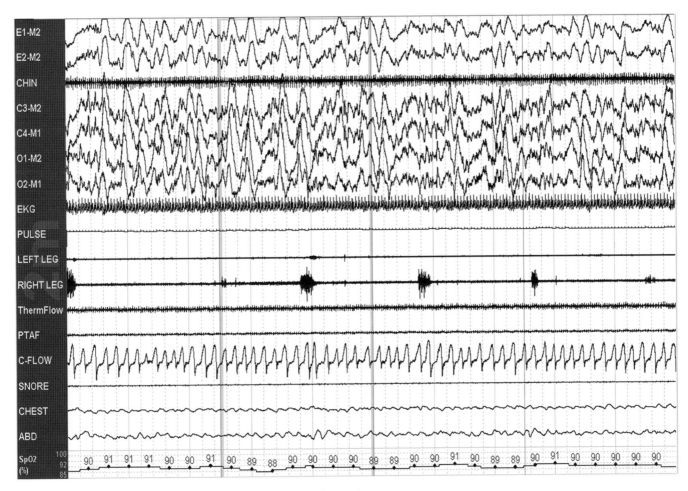

Left Leg, EMG from left leg; Right Leg, EMG from right leg; Spo₂ from pulse oximetry.

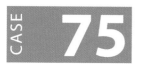

A 62-year-old woman with potential obstructive sleep apnea

Gökhan M. Mutlu and Lisa Wolfe

A 62-year-old woman underwent PSG to assess for OSA. A 30 second epoch from NREM sleep recorded in this patient is shown.

Which of the following statements about the etiology of the EEG and chin EMG findings on this tracing is correct?

A. The prevalence of this sleep disorder increases with age

B. This occurs most commonly during stage N1 and N2 sleep

C. This affects sleep architecture and decreases slow-wave sleep

D. The characteristic feature includes a rhythmic slowing in EEG activity.

Answer on page 182.

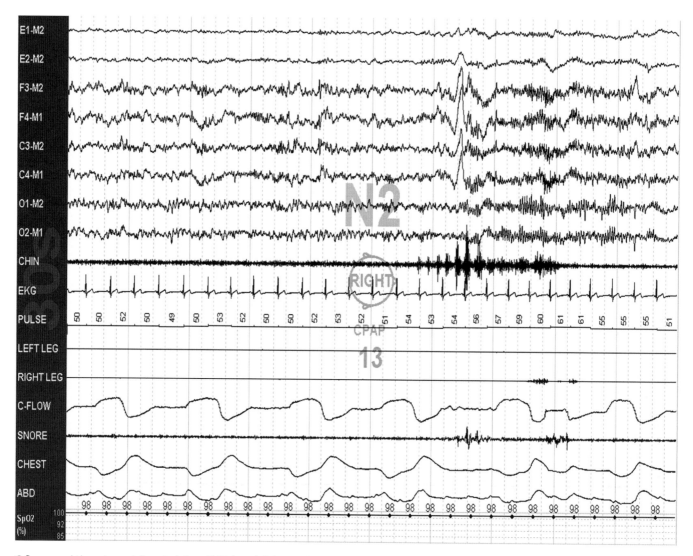

C-flow, nasal thermistor airflow; Left Leg, EMG from left leg; Right Leg, EMG from right leg; CHIN, chin EMG.

Case Studies in Polysomnography Interpretation, ed. Robert C. Basner. Published by Cambridge University Press. © Cambridge University Press 2012.

A 64-year-old morbidly obese man with severe chronic obstructive pulmonary disease and severe obstructive sleep apnea

Gökhan M. Mutlu and Lisa Wolfe

A 64-year-old man with morbid obesity (BMI, 42 kg/m^2), severe COPD and severe OSA (AHI, 48/h) underwent a PAP titration study. He failed to respond to CPAP therapy and bilevel PAP titration was initiated. The events noted in the 30 second epoch below were recorded while on bilevel PAP settings of IPAP/EPAP of 16/13 cmH$_2$O.

What strategy would be most effective to resolve the displayed abnormal finding in the nasal thermistor channel?

A. Increasing IPAP level to augment tidal volume
B. Increasing EPAP level to augment upper airway diameter
C. Addition of a back-up rate of 16 breaths/min to reduce the expiratory time
D. Reducing the sensitivity of the trigger to avoid inappropriate triggering/breath stacking.

Answer on page 183.

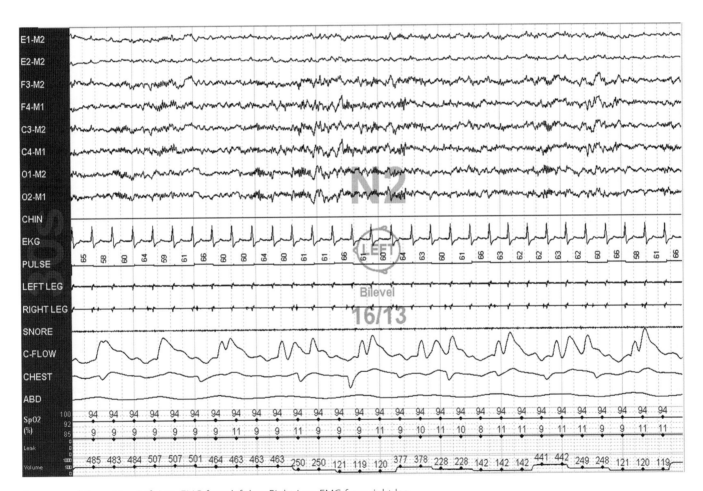

C-flow, nasal thermistor; Left Leg, EMG from left leg; Right Leg, EMG from right leg.

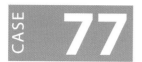

A 30-year-old woman with a diagnosis of moderate obstructive sleep apnea

Gökhan M. Mutlu and Lisa Wolfe

A 30-year-old woman with a diagnosis of moderate OSA underwent CPAP titration. Her past medical history included hypothyroidism, polycystic ovarian syndrome, and dysautonomia. Her medications included desvenlafaxine, trazodone, coenzyme Q10, levocarnitine, and levothyroxine. The patient had a son who developed hypophonia at 4 months of age. He then could not feed and had tongue fasciculations. Metabolic testing was suggestive of mitochondrial disease and genetic testing revealed a mutation in *POLG-1*, encoding mitochondrial DNA polymerase-gamma.

During the titration study, CPAP was unsuccessful because of persistent hypoxemia, and a bilevel PAP titration was initiated. A 2 minute PSG epoch recorded when the patient was on bilevel PAP of IPAP/EPAP of 12/8 cmH₂O is shown.

Which one of the statements below is correct regarding the respiratory abnormality noted in this epoch?

A. This is consistent with Cheyne–Stokes breathing and can be best treated with a servo ventilation device
B. These events are transient, and resolve spontaneously
C. The central apneas are likely caused by a medication
D. The bradypnea/central apnea noted in this study is likely associated with her mitochondrial disease and is best treated with bilevel therapy in spontaneous/timed mode.

Answer on page 184.

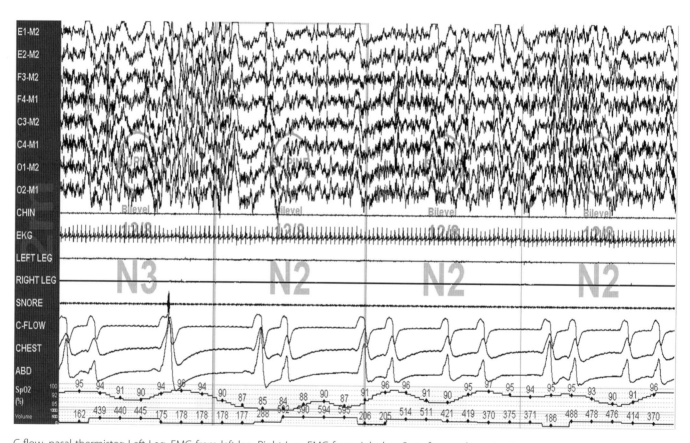

C-flow, nasal thermistor; Left Leg, EMG from left leg; Right Leg, EMG from right leg; SpO₂ from pulse oximetry.

A 75-year-old man with difficulties in initiating sleep and fragmented restless sleep

Irina Ok and Alcibiades Rodriguez

A 75-year-old man presents with difficulties with initiation and maintenance of sleep, and fragmented and restless sleep. He mentions no symptoms at rest. A representative 60 second tracing from his overnight PSG is displayed.

Given this history and this PSG tracing, what is the most likely diagnosis?

A. Restless leg syndrome
B. REM sleep behavior disorder
C. Periodic limb movements of sleep
D. Periodic limb movements of wakefulness.

Answer on page 185.

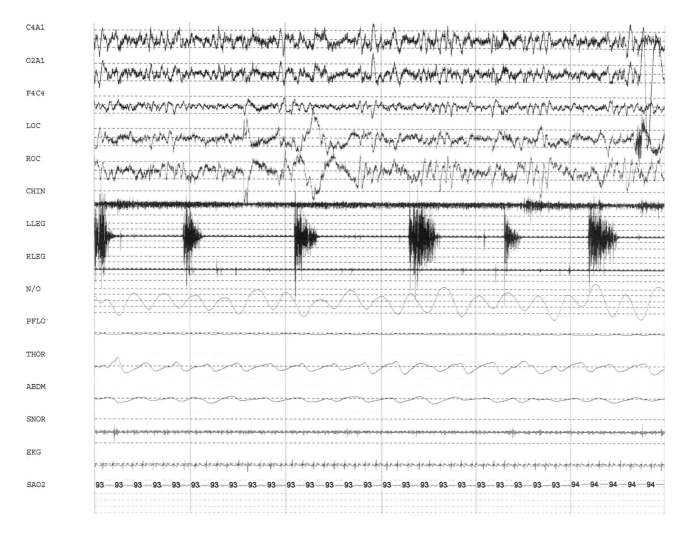

X0.40   60 S   Epoch 855   :   :   Rx:0.0/0.0/0.00

LLEG, Left leg surface EMG; PFLO, nasal pressure transducer (not recorded here).

A 4-year-old girl with mild developmental delay and a history of confusion and abnormal night-time movements of her extremities

Irina Ok and Alcibiades Rodriguez

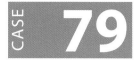

A 4-year-old girl with mild developmental delay presents with a 1 year history of abnormal night-time behavior occurring several times a week. The parents note confusion and some abnormal movements in her extremities. A 30 second epoch from this patient's PSG is shown (Fig. 1).

What does this epoch demonstrate?
A. Normal stage 3 sleep
B. Electrode artifact
C. Bruxism
D. Epileptiform abnormality.

Answer on page 185.

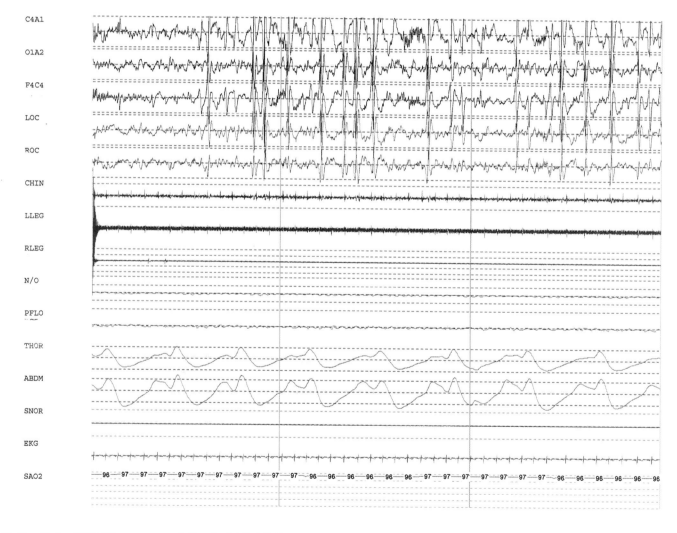

Fig. 1.

A 30-year-old woman with several years of making noises at night and feeling tired

Irina Ok and Alcibiades Rodriguez

A 30-year-old woman presents to the sleep center with several years of making noises at night and feeling tired. She feels that she has not had a restful night of sleep for many years. The only other significant past medical history is evaluation by a dentist and by an ear, nose, and throat physician for facial pain, which they think is related to temporomandibular joint disease. A 30 second epoch is shown from this patient's PSG.

What does this epoch from the PSG show?
A. Bruxism
B. Seizure
C. Arousal
D. Muscle artifact
E. Increased muscle tone during REM sleep.

Answer on page 186.

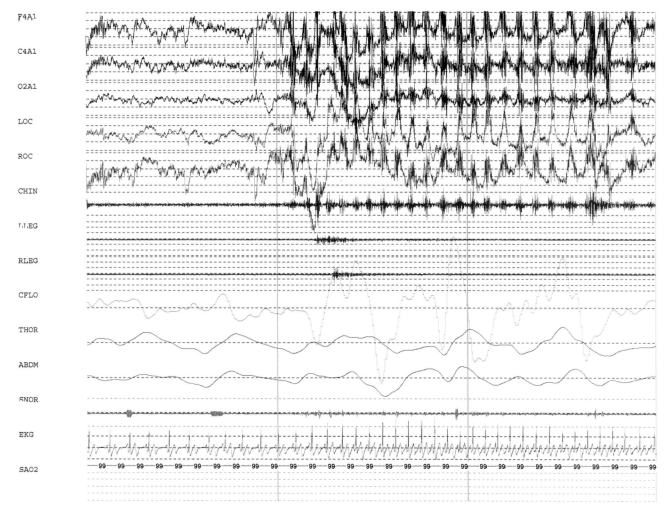

X0.43   30 S   Epoch 508   Back   Rx:0.0/9.0/0.00

CFLO, CPAP channel.

Case Studies in Polysomnography Interpretation, ed. Robert C. Basner. Published by Cambridge University Press. © Cambridge University Press 2012.

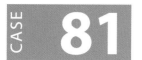

A 35-year-old man with excessive movement of his legs during sleep

Irina Ok and Alcibiades Rodriguez

A 35-year-old man presents with his wife for a consultation related to excessive movement of his legs during sleep. The patient is not aware of this problem, but his wife is concerned that he may have a sleep disorder. There is no significant past medical history.

A 30 second epoch from his PSG is displayed.

Which one of the following is the best interpretation of this PSG tracing?
A. REM sleep
B. Periodic limb movements of sleep
C. Hypnagogic foot tremor
D. Alternating leg muscle activation
E. ECG artifact.

Answer on page 187.

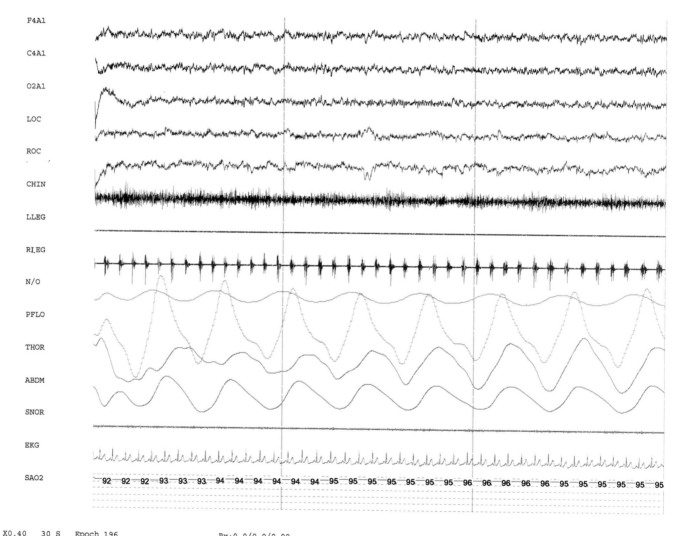

X0.40   30 S   Epoch 196   Rx:0.0/0.0/0.00

A 16-year-old girl with episodes of yelling, crying, and laughing during sleep

Irina Ok and Alcibiades Rodriguez

A 16-year-old girl presents with her mother to a sleep clinic consultation with the chief complaint of abnormal night-time behavior. The patient has developed episodes of yelling, crying, and laughing during sleep, plus, at times, kicking and moving. These episodes occur at least twice a week and are more frequent in the early morning hours. The episodes started after removal of a cavernous angioma from the brainstem approximately 4 months previously.

A 60 second epoch from the patient's PSG is shown.

What is the most compatible explanation for this tracing and history?
A. NREM parasomia
B. REM sleep behavior disorder
C. Seizure
D. Periodic limb movements of sleep.

Answer on page 187.

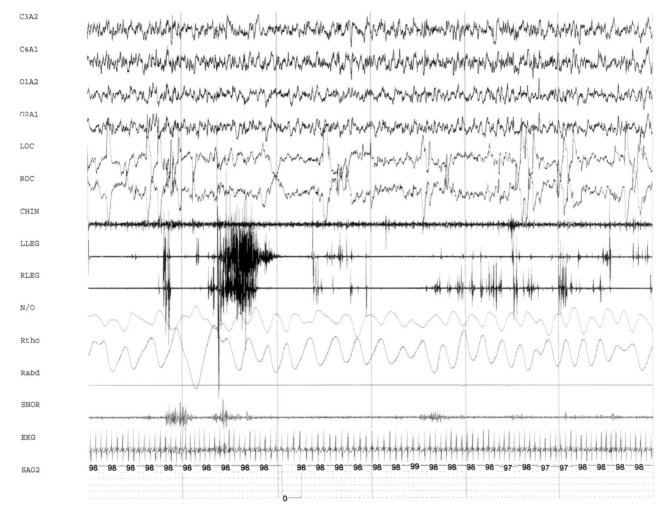

X0.40   60 S   Epoch 396   Rx:0.0/0.0/0.00

Rabd, abdomen respiratory inductance plethysmography; Rtho, thoracic respiratory inductance plethysmography.

Case Studies in Polysomnography Interpretation, ed. Robert C. Basner. Published by Cambridge University Press. © Cambridge University Press 2012.

A 25-year-old woman who bites her tongue during sleep

Irina Ok and Alcibiades Rodriguez

A 25-year-old woman is seen with the chief complaint of waking up with a bitten tongue a couple of times over the past 2 months. She has been placed on clonazepam by a dentist, but she does not remember the reason. There is no other significant past medical history.

A 30 second epoch from her PSG is displayed in Fig. 1.

Which of the following is the best interpretation of this PSG tracing in this setting?

A. Bruxism
B. Normal NREM stage 2 sleep
C. Epileptiform discharges
D. Electrode artifact.

Answer on page 187.

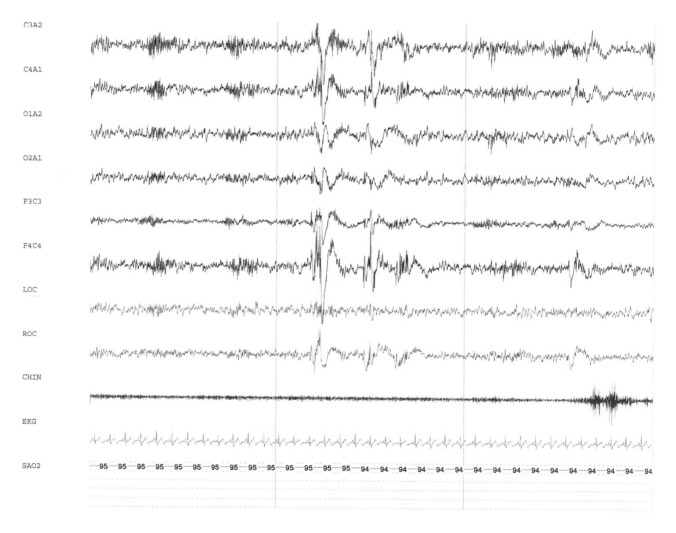

X0.55   30 S   Epoch 1388   Rx:0.0/0.0/0.00

Fig. 1.

A 70-year-old man with abnormal night-time behavior, resulting in falls from the bed

Irina Ok and Alcibiades Rodriguez

A 70-year-old man presented for evaluation to the sleep clinic. He has been experiencing abnormal night-time behavior, which has been getting progressively more frequent over the last few years. He has been in the emergency room twice because of a fall from his bed. He was treated with clonazepam 0.5 mg at bedtime for seizures. However, he had to increase the medication to 2 mg since the behavior was getting worse. His neurologic examination is normal.

The following tracing is a 30 second epoch from his nocturnal PSG.

Based on this history, what is the disorder displayed on the tracing most closely related to?
A. Developmental delay
B. α-Synucleopathy
C. Benzodiazepine use
D. Facial pain
E. Brainstem tumor.

Answer on page 188.

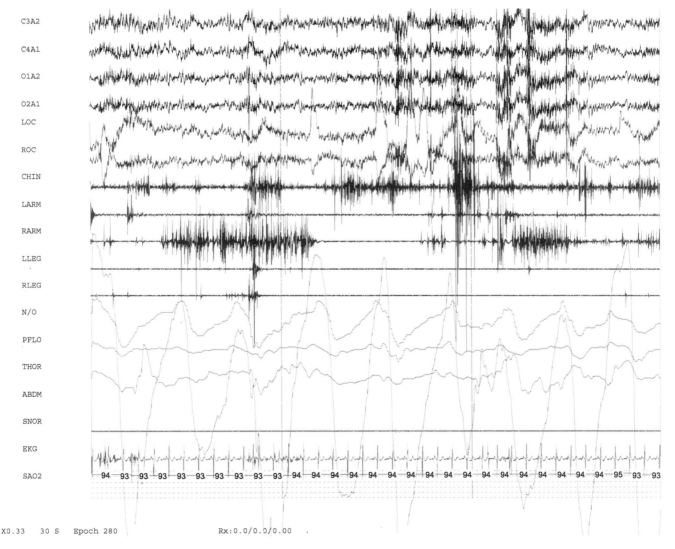

X0.33　30 S　Epoch 280　　　　　Rx:0.0/0.0/0.00

LARM, left arm surface EMG; RARM, right arm surface EMG.

Case Studies in Polysomnography Interpretation, ed. Robert C. Basner. Published by Cambridge University Press. © Cambridge University Press 2012.

A 6-year-old girl with enlarged tonsils and adenoids and a history of snoring and gasping at night

Vidya Pai and Dennis Rosen

A 6-year-old girl with a history of snoring and gasping at night, and with moderately enlarged tonsils and adenoids, was referred for a sleep study to assess for OSA.

The following is a representative 60 second epoch of the PSG.

Based upon this description and interpretation of the representative PSG tracing, what should be recommended as the definitive step in managing this child's condition?

A. Adenotonsillectomy

B. Initiation of bilevel PAP ventilation

C. Obtain an MRI of the brain and brainstem

D. Administration of supplemental O_2 during sleep

E. None of the above.

Answer on page 189.

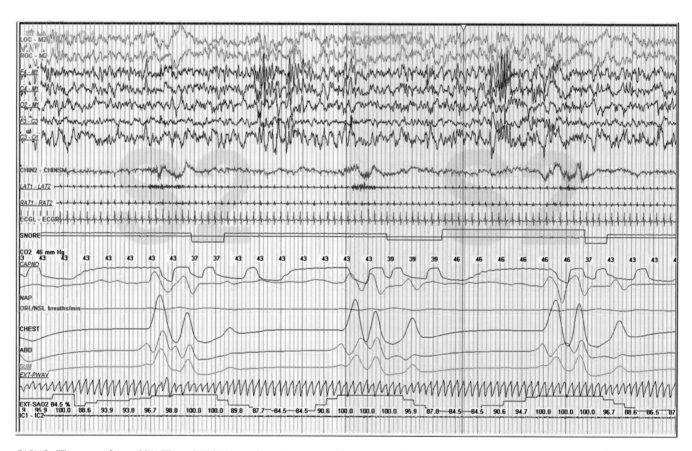

CAPNO, $ETco_2$ waveform; CO2, $ETco_2$; EXT-PWAV, pulse oximeter waveform; IC1–IC2, intercostal EMG; NAP, nasal pressure transducer; ORL/NSL, oronasal thermistor; RAT1–RAT2, right anterior tibialis EMG.

Case Studies in Polysomnography Interpretation, ed. Robert C. Basner. Published by Cambridge University Press. © Cambridge University Press 2012.

A 12-year-old boy with excessive daytime sleepiness

Winnie C. Pao and Timothy I. Morgenthaler

A 12-year-old boy with history significant for mononucleosis, adenotonsillectomy, primary nocturnal enuresis, and increased weight for height (BMI, 30.8 kg/m², which is > 97th percentile) presented with a 1 year history of excessive daytime sleepiness. He snored occasionally but denied any symptoms of restless legs or cataplexy. Examination showed a crowded oropharynx with a Friedman tongue position class III–IV and an elongated uvula. Two weeks of actigraphy demonstrated insufficient total estimated sleep time. A PSG showed an AHI of 1/h (most events occurred in REM sleep while supine), an elevated PLM index (30.5/h), and an arousal index of 17/h, with nearly two thirds of arousals appearing to being movement related. The initial sleep latency was 3.5 minutes; REM latency was 75 minutes, and the sleep efficiency was 88.1%.

Because of the fragmentation associated with PLMs, a serum ferritin level was checked and was 29 µg/L. He was started on iron supplementation and ropinirole for his limb movements. For his positional sleep-disordered breathing, positional therapy was added to a steroid nasal spray, leukotriene inhibitor, and an antihistamine. He returned 2 months later. His serum ferritin level had increased to 50 µg/L, and his BMI had increased to 32.4 kg/m². He continued to feel sleepy during the day, and on repeated questioning endorsed that his face sometimes felt "a little weak" when he laughed. Two weeks of follow-up actigraphy were requested (Fig. 1)

followed by nocturnal PSG (Fig. 2, depicting his typical REM sleep), which was followed by MSLT.

A 16 channel EEG on a second PSG did not show any epileptiform discharges. The AHI was 1/h (3/h in REM). Initial sleep latency was 1 minute, and REM latency was 126 minutes. He slept 483 minutes with a sleep efficiency of 91%. The PLM index was reduced to 16/h (compared with 30.5/h on initial PSG). Sleep remained fragmented, with 17 arousals an hour (one third movement related). Sleep architecture showed a mild increase in slow-wave sleep. The MSLT showed mean sleep latency of 1.13 minutes, and SOREMs in three out of four naps including the fourth nap (nap times were 09:12, 11:05, 13:02, and 15:02). A fifth nap was not assessed after these results were evident.

Based upon the above information and interpretation of the following actigraphy and PSG segments, what is the most accurate primary ICSD-2 diagnosis?
A. Circadian rhythm disorder
B. Periodic limb movement disorder
C. Narcolepsy without cataplexy
D. Idiopathic hypersomnia without long sleep time
E. REM sleep behavior disorder.

Answer on page 190.

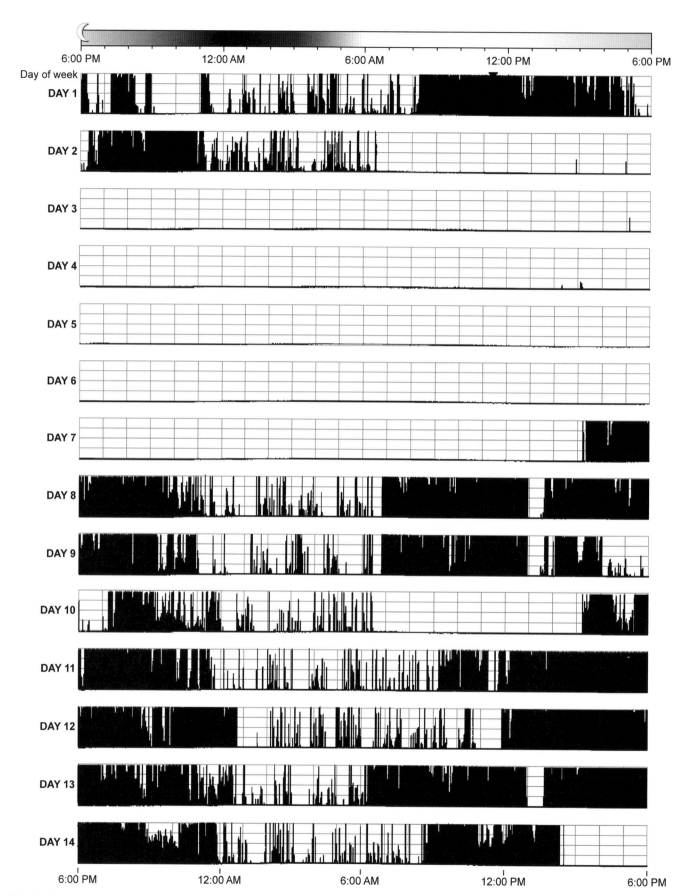

Fig. 1. Actigraphy over 2 weeks.

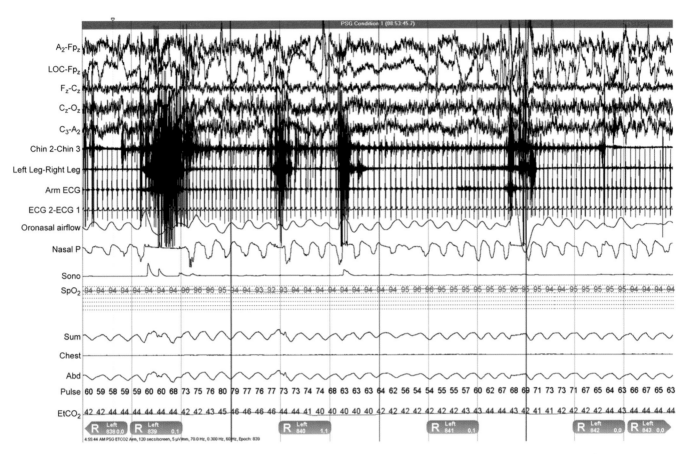

Fig. 2. PSG. A2-Fpz, referential frontal EEG; Chest, thoracic respiratory inductance plethysmography; Leg Leg-Right Leg, pretibial EMG; LOC-Fpz, left referential EOG; Oronasal airflow, thermistor; Spo₂ from pulse oximetry.

A 62-year-old man with congestive heart failure undergoing continuous positive airway pressure titration for obstructive sleep apnea

Nimesh Patel and Sairam Parthasarathy

A 62-year-old man with congestive heart failure is undergoing CPAP titration for OSA, and is noticed to have the following two epochs while receiving CPAP of 8 cmH$_2$O.

1. **Which of the following best describes the respiratory event depicted in the first epoch ("epoch 23") of this tracing?**
   A. Obstructive apnea
   B. Central apnea
   C. Mixed apnea
   D. Complex apnea
   E. Respiratory artifact due to poor belt application
   F. Apnea following bruxism.

2. **Which of the following best describes the oxygen saturation associated with the event defined in the preceding question?**
   A. A desaturation from 94 to 80%
   B. A resaturation from 80 to 96%
   C. A desaturation from 97 to 77%
   D. An association with delayed circulation time
   E. Both C and D
   F. Both B and D
   G. Both A and B.

Answer on page 191.

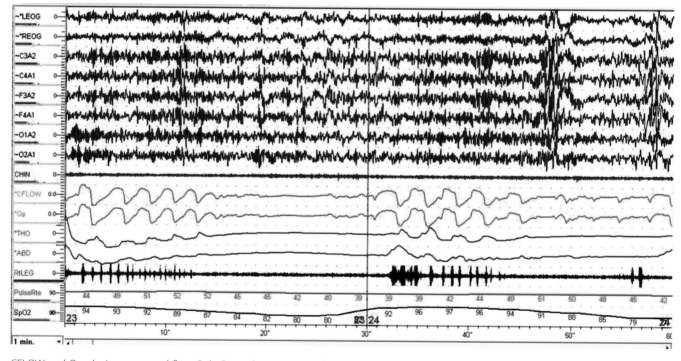

CFLOW and Qp, device-generated flow; PulseRte, pulse rate; RtLEG, leg EMG; Spo$_2$ by finger pulse oximetry; epoch numbers at base. Note that inspiration is positive and exhalation is negative in the flow signals.

Case Studies in Polysomnography Interpretation, ed. Robert C. Basner. Published by Cambridge University Press. © Cambridge University Press 2012.

88

A 54-year-old morbidly obese man with a history of congestive heart failure complaining of loud snoring, excessive daytime sleepiness, fatigue, and nocturia

Nimesh Patel and Sairam Parthasarathy

A 54-year-old morbidly obese man with a history of congestive heart failure complains of loud snoring, excessive daytime sleepiness, fatigue, and nocturia. A nocturnal PSG demonstrates severe OSA and he undergoes PAP titration. The following tracing shows two epochs of this study, which reflect an early point in the study, with the patient receiving bilevel PAP settings of IPAP/EPAP 11/5 cmH$_2$O.

What best describes the respiratory event depicted in the PSG tracing just after the 30 second time point?

A. Obstructive apnea
B. Post-sigh central apnea
C. Mixed apnea
D. Malfunctioning effort belts
E. Normal finding.

Answer on page 192.

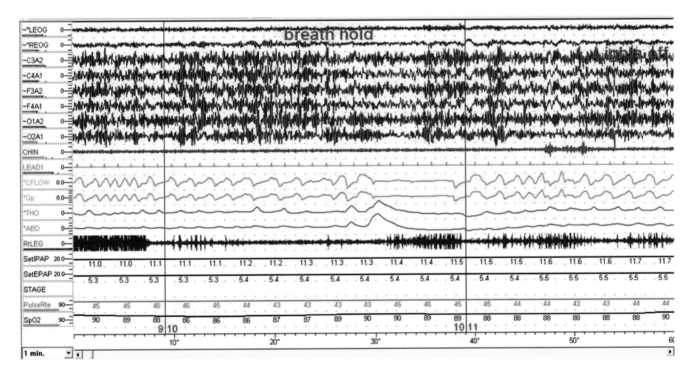

CFLOW and Qp, device-generated flow; RtLEG, leg EMG; setEPAP, EPAP level; setIPAP, IPAP level; Spo$_2$ by finger pulse oximetry; epoch numbers at base. Note that inspiration is positive and exhalation is negative in the flow signals.

A 53-year-old man with history of central sleep apnea and congestive heart failure

Nimesh Patel and Sairam Parthasarathy

A 53-year-old man with history of central sleep apnea and congestive heart failure is noted to have the following four contiguous PSG epochs while receiving servo ventilation. Note that the IPAP (SetIPAP) increases from 26 to 30 cmH$_2$O during the course of the four epochs while the EPAP (SetEPAP) remains steady at 8 cmH$_2$O. The respiratory effort is recorded with non-calibrated respiratory inductance plethysmography belts for thorax and abdomen.

What best describes the respiratory events depicted in the tracing?
A. Obstructive hypopnea
B. Non-obstructive hypopnea
C. Normal breathing
D. Malfunctioning servo ventilation
E. Malfunctioning effort belts.

Answer on page 192.

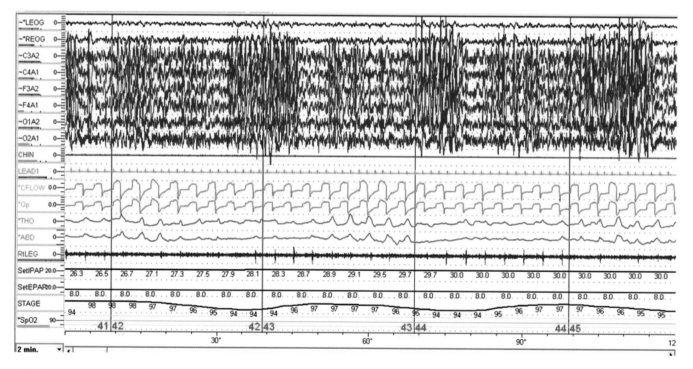

LEAD1, precordial electrocardiogram; Qp, pressure waves derived from CPAP; RtLEG, right EMG; SetEPAP, expiratory pressure; SetIPAP, inspiratory pressure; Spo$_2$ by pulse oximetry.

Case Studies in Polysomnography Interpretation, ed. Robert C. Basner. Published by Cambridge University Press. © Cambridge University Press 2012.

Nimesh Patel and Sairam Parthasarathy

A 33-year-old man with morbid obesity and obesity-hypoventilation syndrome undergoes PSG with volume-assured pressure support ventilation, and has the following consecutive PSG epochs (Fig. 1A,B) recorded early in the study. The patient is supine.

1. What is the sleep stage shown on these tracings?
A. Stage N1
B. Stage N2
C. Stage N3
D. Stage R
E. None of the above; the patient is awake.

2. Does the respiratory response aid in this scoring by AASM criteria?

Answer on page 193.

A

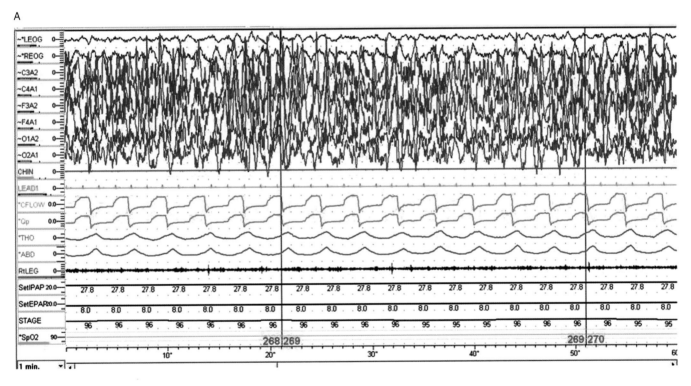

Fig. 1. (A) A 60 second epoch.

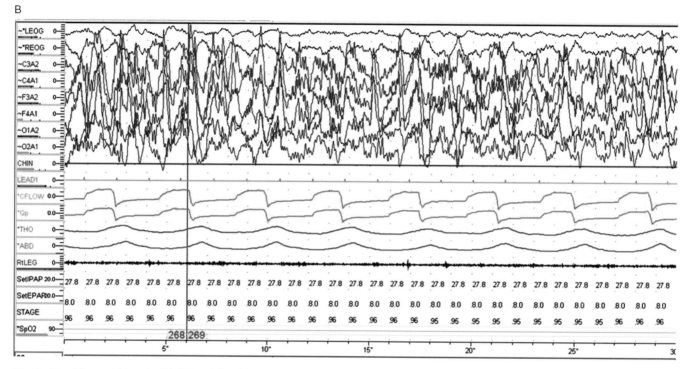

Fig. 1. (B) a 30 second epoch. CFLOW and Qp, device-generated flow; RtLEG, leg EMG; setEPAP, IPAP level; setIPAP, IPAP level; Spo₂ by finger pulse oximetry; epoch numbers at base. Note that inspiration is positive and exhalation is negative in the flow signals.

CASE 91

A 62-year-old man with chronic obstructive pulmonary disease and obstructive sleep apnea

Nimesh Patel and Sairam Parthasarathy

A 62-year-old man with COPD and OSA is undergoing PSG while receiving bilevel PAP ventilation. The patient's sleep-disordered breathing is effectively controlled until he develops the following series of epochs.

Based upon interpretation of this tracing, what is the likely cause of the oxygen desaturation in the epochs shown?

A. Stage R

B. Ventilation–perfusion mismatch

C. Hypoventilation

D. Air leak

E. All of the above.

Answer on page 193.

Case Studies in Polysomnography Interpretation, ed. Robert C. Basner. Published by Cambridge University Press. © Cambridge University Press 2012.

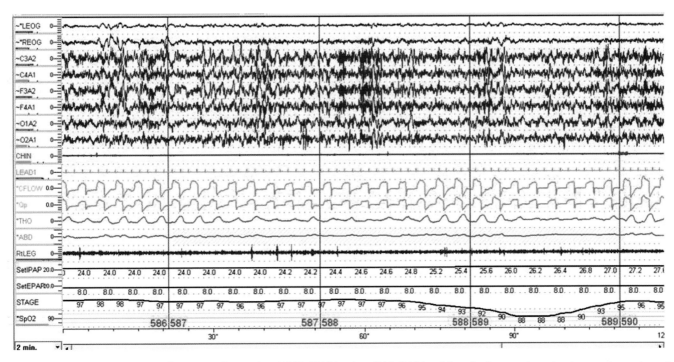

CFLOW and Qp, device-generated flow; RtLEG, leg EMG; setEPAP, EPAP level; setIPAP, IPAP level; Spo₂ by finger pulse oximetry; epoch numbers at base. Note that inspiration is positive and exhalation is negative in the flow signals.

CASE 92

A 56-year-old woman who smokes and is obese

Sachin R. Pendharkar and W. Ward Flemons

The following tracing is a 120 second epoch of REM sleep from a "split-night" PSG study of a 56-year-old woman who smokes and is obese. She presents with excessive daytime sleepiness. (Room air arterial blood gas parameters are pH 7.40, $Paco_2$ 48 mmHg, Pao_2 60 mmHg, HCO_3 30 mmol/L, Spo_2 82%, P_{bar}, 660 torr.) Baseline transcutaneous Pco_2 ($TCco_2$) is 47 mmHg.

Based on interpretation of the PSG epoch shown, and this history, what is the most appropriate initial treatment regimen?
A. Continuous positive airway pressure
B. Therapy with CPAP and O_2
C. Bilevel PAP
D. Servo ventilation
E. Oxygen alone.

Answer on page 194.

Case Studies in Polysomnography Interpretation, ed. Robert C. Basner. Published by Cambridge University Press. © Cambridge University Press 2012.

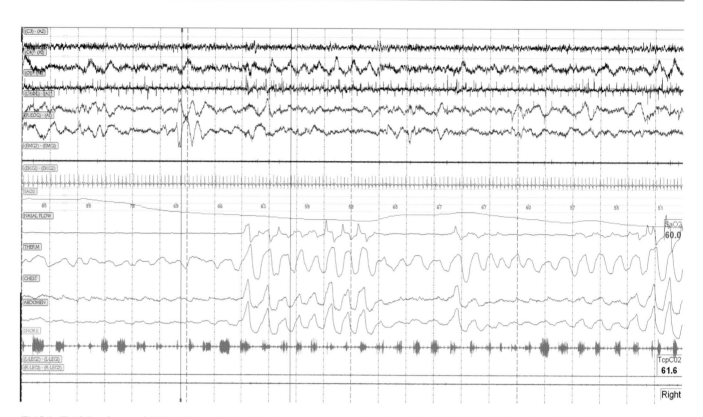

(EMG1)–(EMG2), submental EMG; HCO₃, calculated bicarbonate concentration (mmol/L); (L-LEG2)–(L-LEG1), left leg EMG; NASAL FLOW, pneumotachograph nasal flow sensor; P_bar, barometric pressure; (R-LEG1)–(R-LEG2), right leg EMG; THERM, oronasal thermistor.

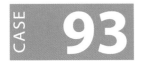

A 76-year-old man with exertional dyspnea, orthopnea and excessive daytime sleepiness

Sachin R. Pendharkar and W. Ward Flemons

A 76-year-old man is complaining of exertional dyspnea, orthopnea and excessive daytime sleepiness. His BMI is 27 kg/m². (Room air awake arterial blood gas parameters are pH 7.40, $Paco_2$ 45 mmHg, Pao_2 68 mmHg, HCO_3 27 mmol/L, Spo_2 93%, and P_{bar} 660 torr.) Baseline awake $TCco_2$ is 46 mmHg. Oxygen was added for hypoxemia in REM sleep. The technologist indicated that all signals are working normally. The following are 120 second epochs, in stage N2 sleep (A) and in REM sleep (B).

Based on this history and interpretation of these PSG tracings, what is the most likely diagnosis?
A. Obstructive sleep apnea
B. Obesity-hypoventilation syndrome
C. Spinal cord injury at the level of T3
D. Diaphragmatic weakness
E. Cheyne–Stokes breathing.

Answer on page 195.

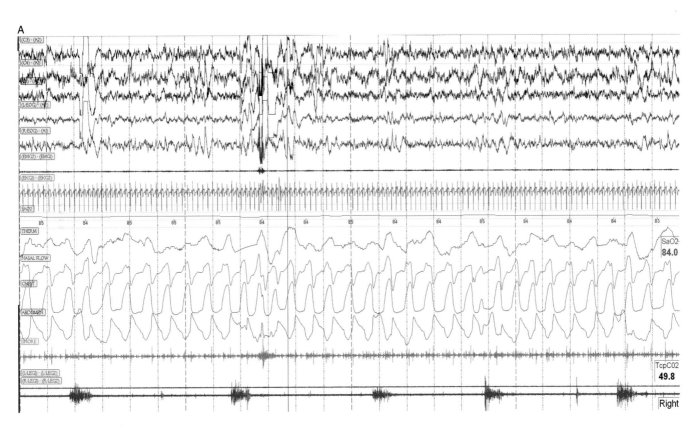

Fig. 1. (A) stage N2 sleep.

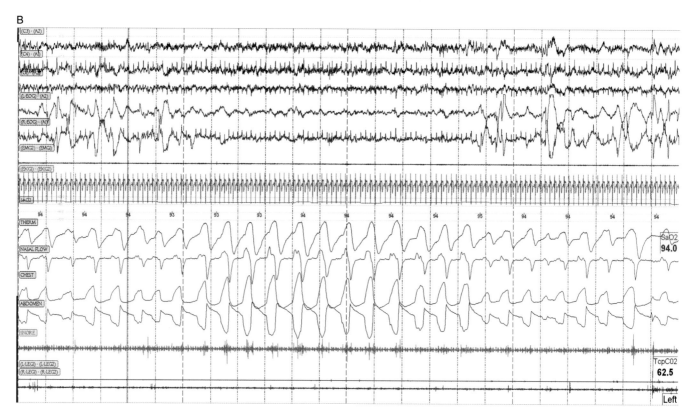

Fig. 1. (B) REM sleep. (EMG1)–(EMG2), submental EMG; HCO₃, calculated bicarbonate concentration (mmol/L); (L-LEG2)–(L-LEG1), left leg EMG; NASAL FLOW, pneumotachograph nasal flow sensor; P_bar, barometric pressure; (R-LEG1)–(R-LEG2), right leg EMG; N2, AASM stage N2 sleep; THERM, oronasal thermistor; SAO2, Spo₂ by finger pulse oximetry.

A 63-year-old man with snoring, witnessed apnea, fragmented nocturnal sleep, and daytime sleepiness

Bharati Prasad

A 63-year-old man has snoring, witnessed apnea, fragmented nocturnal sleep, and daytime sleepiness, without any known cardiopulmonary disease. The following is a continuous 5 minute PSG tracing in this patient.

What is the best interpretation for the respiratory findings observed during continuous positive airway pressure titration in this "split-night" study?

A. Primary central sleep apnea
B. Cheyne–Stokes breathing
C. Periodic limb movement arousals
D. Complex sleep apnea.

Answer on page 196.

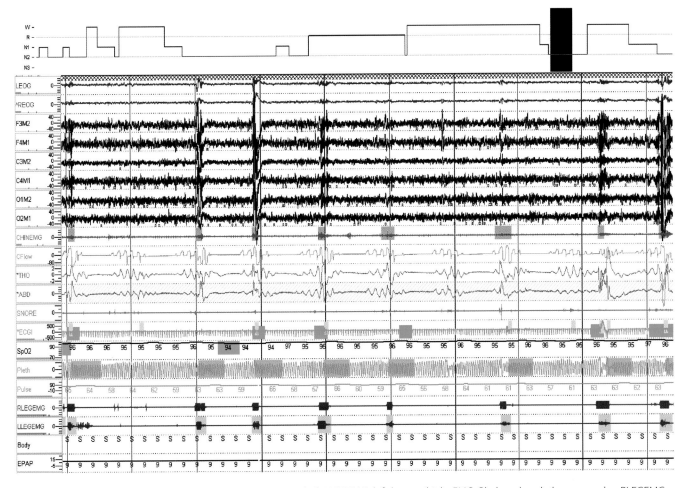

Body, body position; EPAP, CPAP minus expiratory pressure relief; LLEGEMG, left lower tibialis EMG; Pleth, pulse plethysmography; RLEGEMG, right lower tibialis EMG.

A 60-year-old woman with a history of moderate snoring and witnessed pauses in breathing plus long-term insomnia

Stuart F. Quan

A 60-year-old woman presents with a history of moderate snoring and witnessed pauses in breathing for several years. In addition, she has difficulty initiating sleep and has frequent nocturnal arousals. She has had the insomnia symptoms most of her life, but these have worsened over the past several months. She feels fatigued but not sleepy during the day. Recently, the patient has been sleep-talking and moving her arms and legs in her sleep. There have been no injuries because of her body movements, but they occur nightly and her husband now sleeps in a separate room. She has no recollection of the events. Her past medical history includes migraine headaches, arthritis, depression, and anxiety. The patient is taking paroxetine and propranolol. Physical examination is remarkable only for mild obesity (BMI 31 kg/m^2). A PSG was ordered with the following results:

total recording time: 381.0 minutes
total sleep time: 324.5 minutes
sleep efficiency: 85.2%
sleep latency: 8 minutes
AHI: 22.7/h
N1: 15.9%

N2: 56.7%
N3: 0%
REM: 27.4%
PLM index: 20/h.

Figure 1 is an epoch from the PSG. At the time midway in the tracing shown, the technician noted that "the patient jumped in her sleep in a startle response and 'yelped'".

Figure 2 is a representative epoch from the same PSG during REM sleep.

Based on this information and the interpretation of the displayed PSGs, what is the best initial treatment for this patient?
A. Discontinue propranolol
B. Discontinue paroxetine
C. Begin clonazepam
D. Begin pramipexole
E. Begin autoPAP.

Answer on page 196.

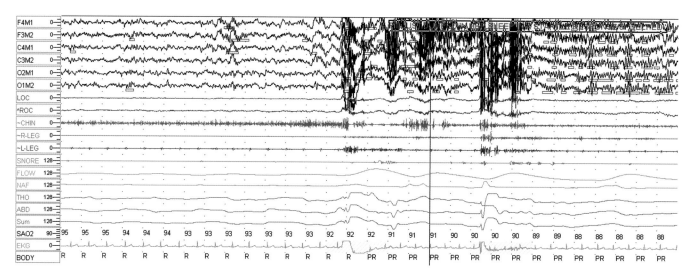

Fig. 1. BODY, body position; Flow, airflow from oronasal thermistor; SAo$_2$ from pulse oximetry.

Case Studies in Polysomnography Interpretation, ed. Robert C. Basner. Published by Cambridge University Press. © Cambridge University Press 2012.

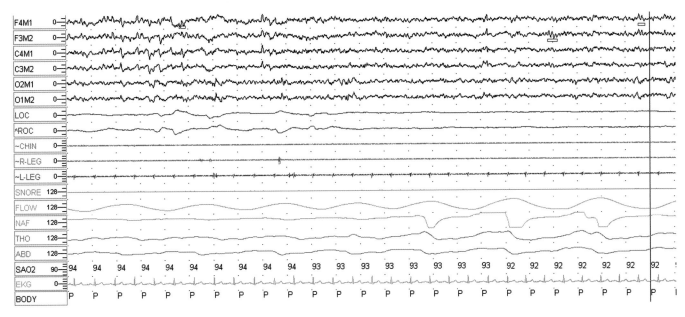

Fig. 2. BODY, body position; Flow, airflow from oronasal thermistor.

A 55-year-old woman with daytime fatigue and unrefreshing sleep of several years' duration

Stuart F. Quan

The following two discontinuous 30 second PSG epochs were recorded from a 55-year-old woman who presented with daytime fatigue and unrefreshing sleep of several years duration.

Which of the following conditions is commonly associated with the finding observed in these epochs?

A. Obstructive sleep apnea

B. Fibromyalgia

C. Chronic benzodiazepine use

D. Periodic limb movement disorder

Answer on page 197.

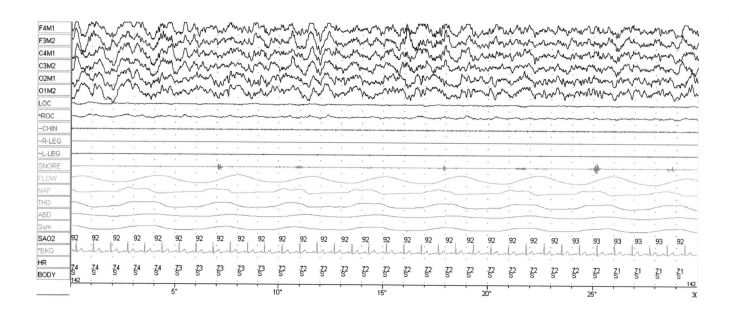

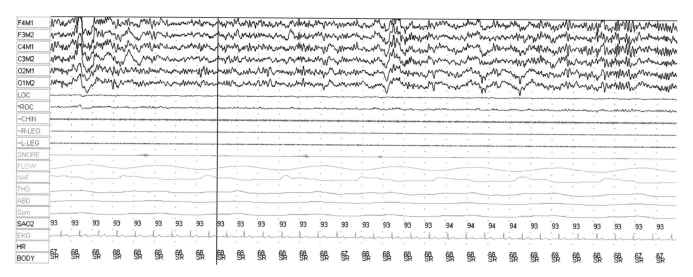

BODY, body position; Flow, airflow from oronasal thermistor.

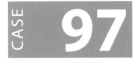

An 8-year-old child with profound developmental delay and intractable seizures being treated with antiepileptic medications and an implanted vagal nerve stimulator

Dennis Rosen

An 8-year-old child with profound developmental delay and intractable seizures who was being treated with antiepileptic medications recently underwent implantation of a vagal nerve stimulator. He is now referred for a sleep study to assess for possible sleep-disordered breathing. Two PSG tracings from this study are displayed. Figure 1A is a 120 second epoch; Fig. 1B is a 60 second epoch.

While no overt obstructive or central sleep apnea was noted, very frequent episodes of attenuation of the nasal thermistor airflow signal (Oral/NSL) occurred. Examples of this can be seen within the portions of the tracings demarcated by black arrows. The electrical activity of the vagal nerve stimulator was recorded on the bottom channel of the montage and is underlined in red.

A

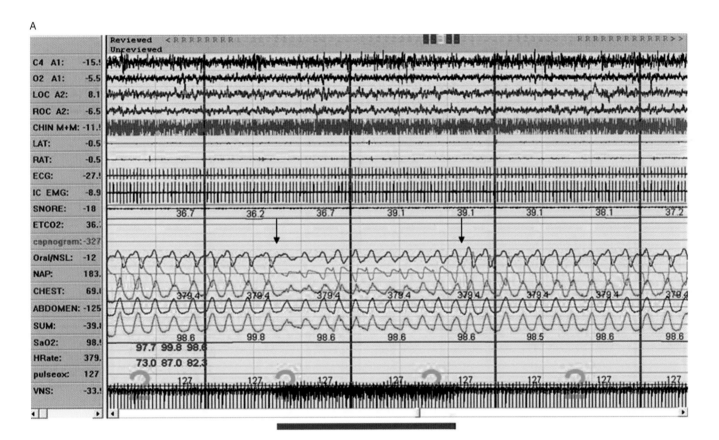

Fig. 1. (A) A 120 second epoch.

B

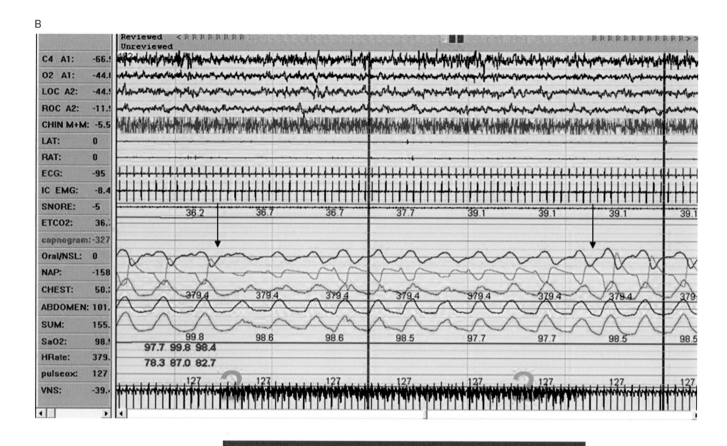

Fig. 1. (B) a 60 second epoch. IC EMG, intercostal EMG; NAP, nasal pressure transducer; Oral/NSL, oronasal thermistor; pulseox, pulse oximetry signal; RAT, right anterior tibialis EMG; VNS, vagal nerve stimulator.

What is the best interpretation for the frequent decreases in airflow on these PSG tracings as measured by the nasal thermistor?

A. Seizure activity compromising respiratory effort
B. Obstructive hypopneas

C. Decreased respiratory effort secondary to the vagal nerve stimulator activity
D. Central sleep apneas.

Answer on page 198.

A 9-year-old girl with a history of snoring, gasping, and chronic mouth breathing

Dennis Rosen

A 9-year-old girl with moderate size tonsils and adenoids was referred to the sleep laboratory for a sleep study to rule out OSA because of a history of snoring, gasping, and chronic mouth breathing. Upon review of her study, she was noted to have frequent discharges on the leg EMG recordings; no movements were seen on the video recording. These discharges were seen in all sleep stages, and none resulted in arousal. They were noted across almost the entire sleep night. Two screenshots from the study are presented; Fig. 1A shows a 60 second epoch and Fig. 1B is a 10 second epoch. The discharges are marked with black arrows.

What is the best interpretation of the EMG discharges displayed?

A. Periodic limb movements of sleep
B. Movement secondary to respiratory disturbance
C. Hypnagogic foot tremor
D. Excessive fragmentary myoclonus.

Answer on page 198.

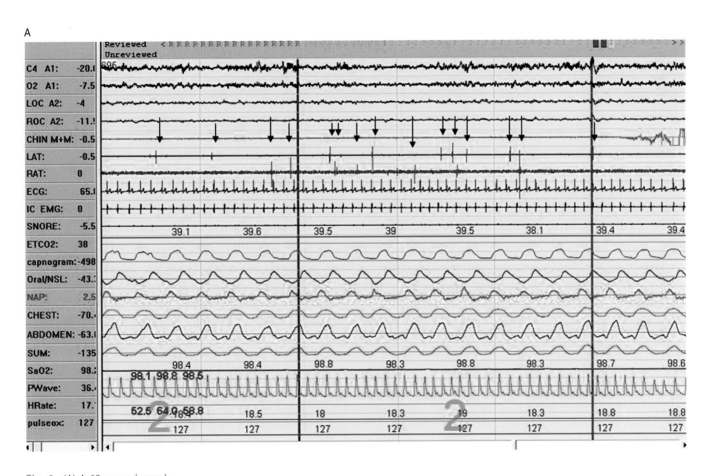

Fig. 1. (A) A 60 second epoch.

B

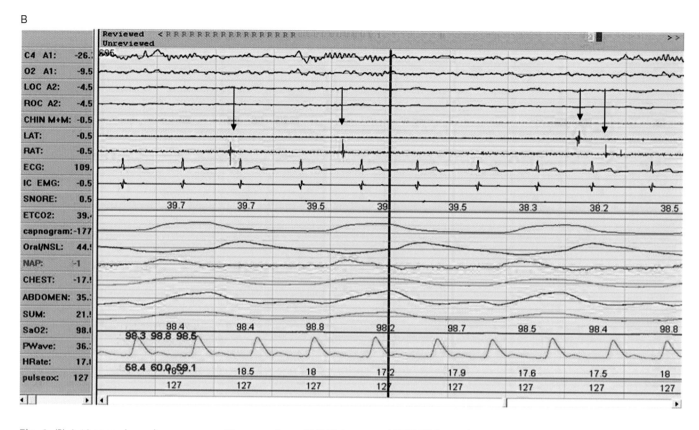

Fig. 1. (B) A 10 second epoch. capnogram, ETco$_2$ waveform; IC EMG, intercostal EMG; NAP, nasal pressure transducer; Oral/NSL, oronasal thermistor; pulseox, pulse oximetry signal; PWave, pulse waveform.

A 42-year-old obese man with worsening snoring and excessive daytime sleepiness

Vijay Seelall

A 42-year-old man is seen in the sleep center because his wife has noted worsening snoring over the past few years. The patient has also noted excessive daytime sleepiness over this period but attributes this to his busy work schedule and associated insufficient sleep. His BMI is 31 kg/m^2. His wife notes that his snoring is worse in the supine position, and when he drinks alcohol. He undergoes nocturnal PSG. A representative 2 minute PSG tracing from this study, with the patient supine, is shown.

Based on this history and interpretation of this representative PSG tracing, what should be the next therapy for this patient?
A. Continuous positive airway pressure
B. Radiofrequency palate surgery
C. Positional therapy and weight loss
D. Zolpidem.

Answer on page 199.

Case Studies in Polysomnography Interpretation, ed. Robert C. Basner. Published by Cambridge University Press. © Cambridge University Press 2012.

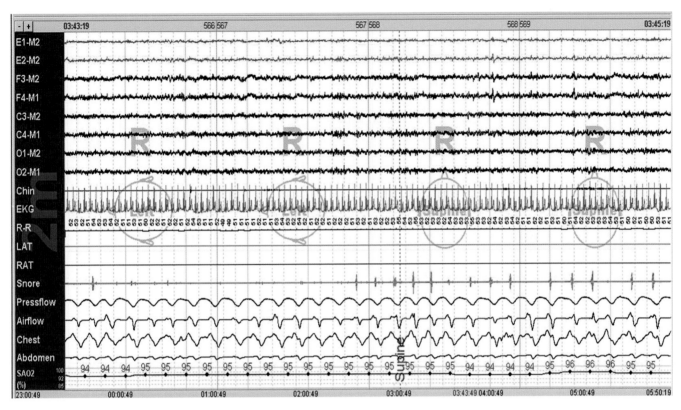

Abdomen, abdominal respiratory inductance plethysmography; Airflow, oronasal thermistor; Chest, thoracic respiratory inductance plethysmography; Pressflow, nasal pressure transducer; R-R, pulse rate from pulse oximetry.

100 A 67-year-old man with class III heart failure

Vijay Seelall

The following 5 minute PSG tracing is from a 67-year-old man with New York Heart Association functional class III heart failure. The tracing is representative of the patient's full overnight PSG.

Based on this history and interpretation of this representative PSG tracing, which of the following is correct regarding this patient's sleep-related breathing disorder?

A. Use of CPAP has not been shown to improve survival in this setting

B. Risk factors for this type of sleep-disordered breathing in patients with heart failure include male gender, advanced age, atrial fibrillation and hypercapnia

C. This type of sleep-disordered breathing in this setting is associated with a worse prognosis than the absence of such sleep-disordered breathing

D. Periodic limb movements in sleep are scored in association with the central apneas.

Answer on page 199.

Case Studies in Polysomnography Interpretation, ed. Robert C. Basner. Published by Cambridge University Press. © Cambridge Universty Press 2012.

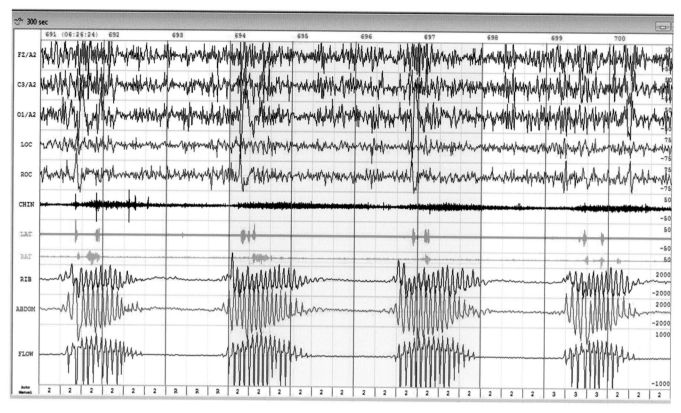

FZ/A2, frontal referential EEG; Rib, thoracic respiratory inductance plethysmography.

CASE 101

A 62-year-old obese man with hypertension, diastolic dysfunction, mild aortic stenosis, and paroxysmal atrial fibrillation

Anita Valanju Shelgikar

The following 1 minute PSG tracing was recorded in a 62-year-old man with obesity, hypertension, grade 1 diastolic dysfunction, mild aortic stenosis, and paroxysmal atrial fibrillation.

What is the best interpretation of the ECG during the first and second portions of the tracing?

A. Normal sinus rhythm, followed by normal sinus rhythm
B. Normal sinus rhythm, followed by wide complex tachycardia
C. Sinus tachycardia, followed by atrial fibrillation
D. Normal sinus rhythm, followed by atrial fibrillation
E. Sinus tachycardia, followed by first-degree AV block.

Answer on page 200.

Case Studies in Polysomnography Interpretation, ed. Robert C. Basner. Published by Cambridge University Press. © Cambridge University Press 2012.

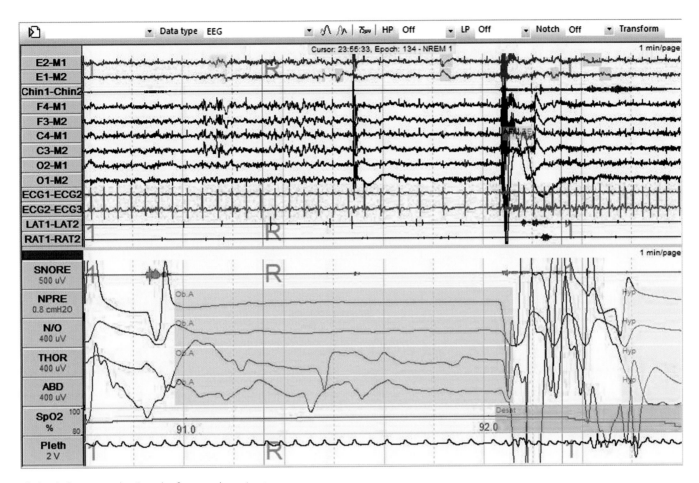

Pleth, plethysmography; Spo$_2$ by finger pulse oximetry.

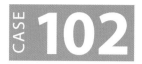

CASE 102

A 45-year-old man with a history of snoring, morning headaches, and excessive daytime somnolence

Jeffrey J. Stanley and Judy Fetterolf

A 45-year-old man with a history of snoring, morning headaches and excessive daytime somnolence underwent diagnostic PSG. A representative 30 second epoch from his overnight PSG is shown.

What is the best interpretation of the type of artifact present on the PSG tracing?

A. ECG artifact

B. A 60 Hz artifact

C. Electrode popping

D. Sweat artifact.

Answer on page 200.

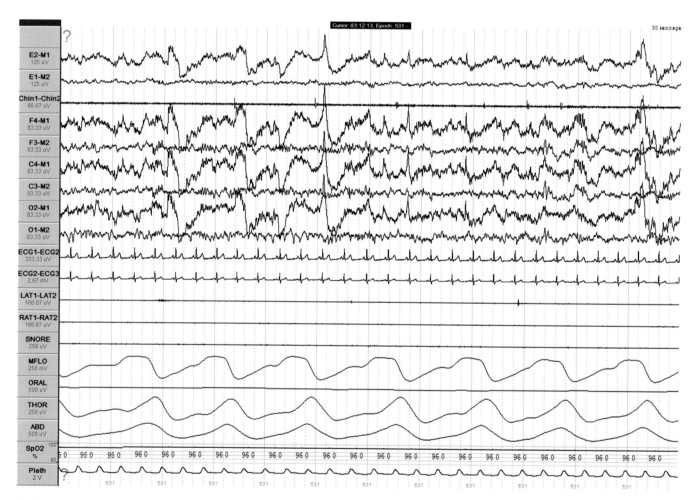

Pleth, pulse rate from pulse oximeter; Spo₂ by pulse oximetry.

103 A morbidly obese 3-year-old boy with a history of loud snoring and witnessed apneic episodes

Jeffrey J. Stanley and Judy Fetterolf

A morbidly obese 3-year-old boy with a history of very loud ("heroic") snoring and witnessed apneic episodes underwent diagnostic PSG. A representative 30 second tracing from his overnight PSG is shown.

What is the best interpretation of the type of artifact present on the PSG tracing?

A. ECG artifact
B. A 60 Hz artifact
C. Electrode popping
D. Sweat artifact.

Answer on page 201.

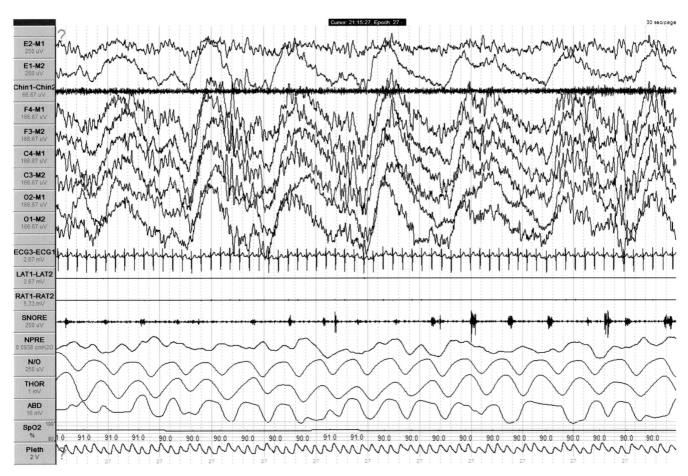

Pleth, pulse rate from pulse oximeter; Spo₂ by pulse oximetry.

Case Studies in Polysomnography Interpretation, ed. Robert C. Basner. Published by Cambridge University Press. © Cambridge University Press 2012.

Jeffrey J. Stanley and Judy Fetterolf

A 59-year-old man with a history of coronary artery disease and excessive daytime somnolence underwent diagnostic PSG to assess for a sleep-related breathing disorder. Two representative tracings from his overnight PSG, each 30 seconds, are shown.

What is the most accurate interpretation of the type of artifact present on each of the PSG tracings?

A. ECG artifact
B. A 60 Hz artifact
C. Electrode popping
D. Sweat artifact
E. Interictal seizure focus.

Answer on page 201.

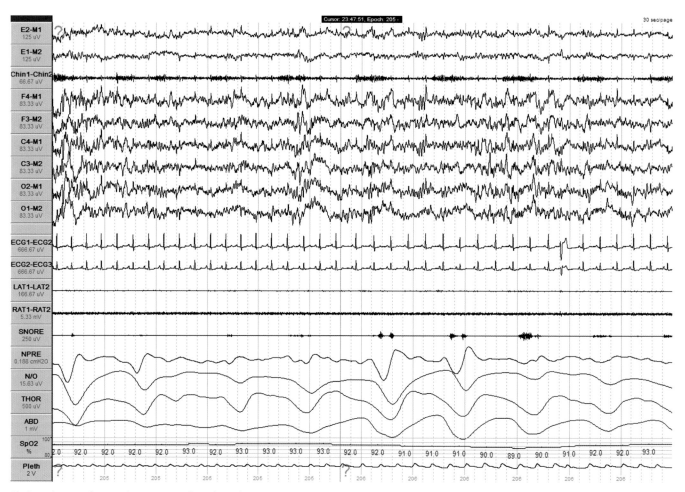

Pleth, pulse rate from pulse oximeter; Spo$_2$ by pulse oximetry.

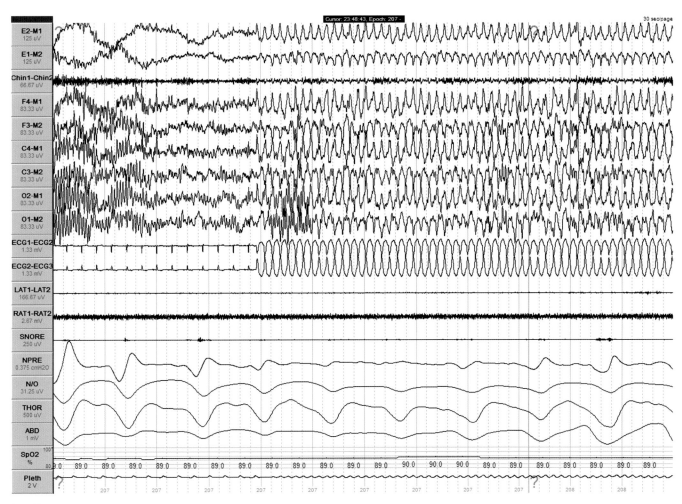

(cont.)

An 18-year-old woman treated for narcolepsy with cataplexy

Shannon S. Sullivan and Christian Guilleminault

An 18-year-old woman has been treated at a sleep disorders center for narcolepsy with cataplexy. She presents now with continued excessive daytime sleepiness despite alerting medications, adequate total sleep time, and scheduled naps. She undergoes nocturnal PSG and is found to have sleep-disordered breathing; she subsequently is referred for a CPAP titration. An approximately 30 second tracing from this PSG is shown (Fig. 1); the patient is being treated with 11 cmH$_2$O CPAP at the time of the tracing.

1. **What medication used in narcolepsy with cataplexy may be associated with an increase in the activity shown in the PSG?**
A. Amphetamine
B. Clomipramine
C. Gamma hydroxybutyrate
D. Atomoxetine
E. Venlafaxine.

During the overnight PSG, the patient has difficulty adjusting to the CPAP mask, complaining of claustrophobia. Within several hours of sleep onset, she stirs and sits up in bed, as shown in the following approximately 105 second PSG tracing (Fig. 2; still with 11 cmH$_2$O CPAP).

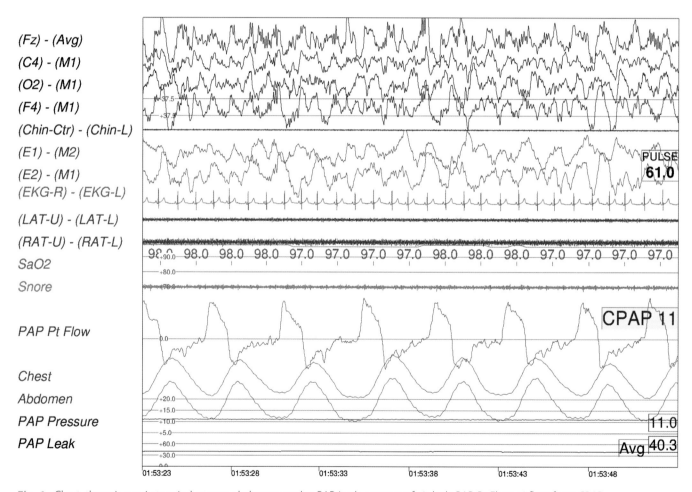

Fig. 1. Chest, thoracic respiratory inductance plethysmography; PAP Leak, amount of air leak; PAP Pt Flow, airflow from CPAP.

Case Studies in Polysomnography Interpretation, ed. Robert C. Basner. Published by Cambridge University Press. © Cambridge University Press 2012.

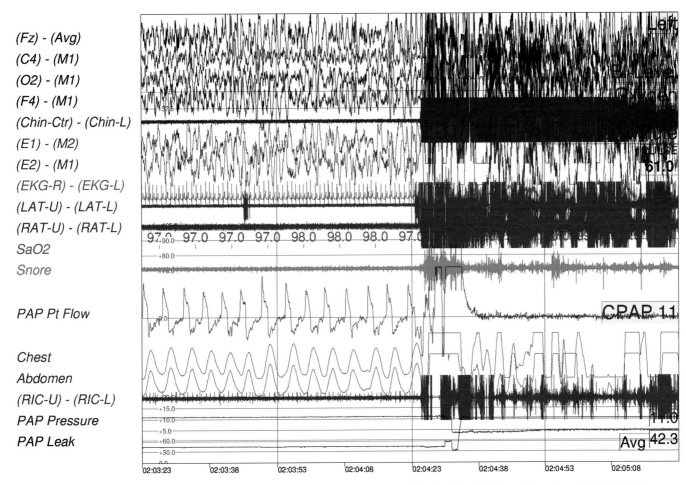

(Fz) - (Avg)
(C4) - (M1)
(O2) - (M1)
(F4) - (M1)
(Chin-Ctr) - (Chin-L)
(E1) - (M2)
(E2) - (M1)
(EKG-R) - (EKG-L)
(LAT-U) - (LAT-L)
(RAT-U) - (RAT-L)
SaO2
Snore

PAP Pt Flow

Chest
Abdomen
(RIC-U) - (RIC-L)
PAP Pressure
PAP Leak

Fig. 2. Chest, thoracic respiratory inductance plethysmography; PAP Leak, amount of air leak; PAP Pt Flow, airflow from CPAP; RIC, right intercostal EMG.

She is disoriented, exhibits slow speech, and has a blunted response to the sleep technologist who comes to assist her; she resists when assistance is attempted. She fumbles to remove the EEG, EOG, and other PSG leads. After about 10 minutes she lies down and the remainder of the night is uneventful. In the morning she does not recall the event.

2. What is the best interpretation of the event in light of the description given?
A. REM sleep behavior disorder
B. Sleep terror
C. Somnambulism
D. Confusional arousal
E. Nightmare disorder.

Answer on page 202.

A 20-year-old man with a history of inappropriate night-time behavior

Shannon S. Sullivan and Christian Guilleminault

A 20-year-old man presents to the sleep clinic with a history of inappropriate night-time behavior. This usually occurs after about 1–2 hours of sleep, and happens two to three times per month. There is no history of stereotyped behavior. He undergoes PSG during a holiday break, having just completed his final examinations. After 100 minutes, he sits up in bed and cries out loudly; he appears frantic. He is sweaty and his heart rate increases. He does not awaken when the sleep technologist comes to assist him; rather, he becomes more agitated and resistive. The event lasts 5 minutes and he has no recollection in the morning. The following PSG tracing shows the episode.

Based on this description and the representative PSG tracing, how is this event best described?
A. Sleep terror
B. Confusional arousal
C. Sleep-walking
D. Nightmare
E. REM sleep behavior disorder.

Answer on page 202.

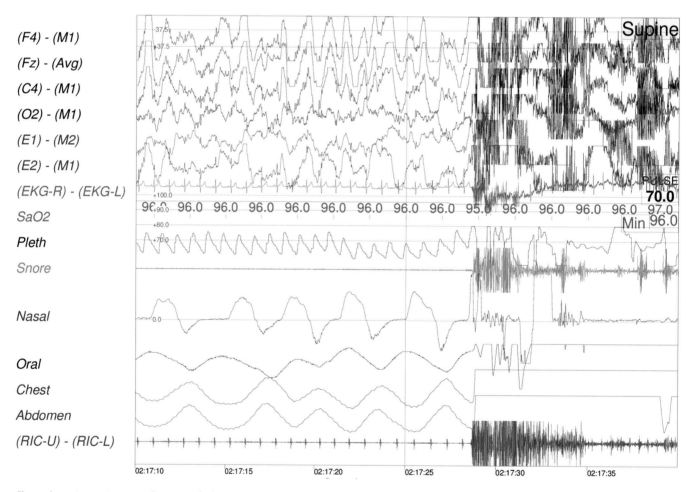

Chest, thoracic respiratory inductance plethysmography; Nasal, nasal pressure transducer; Oral, oronasal thermistor; Pleth, finger photoplethysmography; RIC, right intercostal EMG.

An otherwise healthy college student with an isolated incident of abnormal nocturnal behavior

Shannon S. Sullivan and Christian Guilleminault

An otherwise healthy college student is referred to the sleep clinic to work up an isolated incident of abnormal nocturnal behavior. Two weeks before, after consuming four beers at a party marking the end of final examinations, he returned to his dormitory room and lay on the bed for 2 hours. He then rose from bed and urinated in the corner of the room. When his roommate attempted to stop him, he was poorly responsive; with further attempts to restrain him, he became aggressive and pushed his roommate to the floor. He did not recall the event in the morning. History reveals snoring three to four nights per week and chronic sleep restriction related to busy academic, sport, and work schedules. Nocturnal PSG is performed but does not reveal any of the abnormal behavior

described. A representative approximately 60 second tracing from that PSG is shown.

Based on the history and interpretation of the PSG tracing, what is the best next step in treatment?
A. Referral to neurology for nocturnal seizure disorder
B. Referral to behavioral therapy for anger management
C. Clonazepam for RBD
D. Treat OSA, alcohol counseling, and sleep hygiene
E. Nothing; this type of event is common in the population and generally requires no treatment.

Answer on page 203.

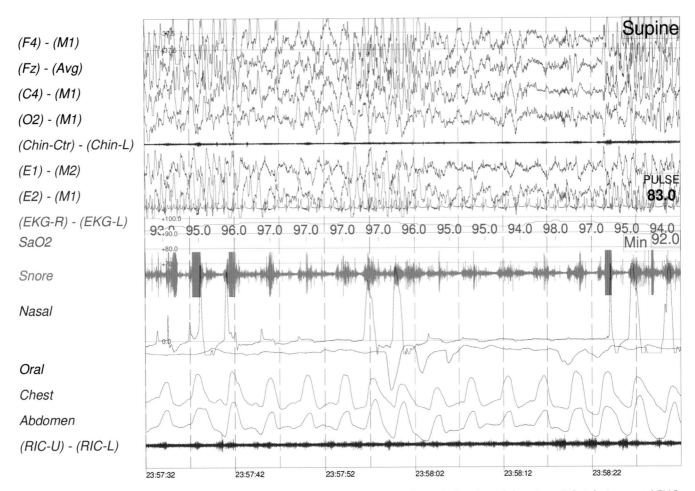

Chest, thoracic respiratory inductance plethysmography; Nasal, nasal pressure transducer; Oral, oral nasal thermistor; RIC, right intercostal EMG.

Case Studies in Polysomnography Interpretation, ed. Robert C. Basner. Published by Cambridge University Press. © Cambridge University Press 2012.

A 52-year-old man with amyotrophic lateral sclerosis, excessive sleepiness, and early morning headache

Peter J.-C. Wu and John R. Wheatley

A 52-year-old man was referred to the respiratory clinic for the assessment of sleepiness. He had been diagnosed with amyotrophic lateral sclerosis a year before, with predominantly lower limb involvement. There was minimal bulbar involvement. The patient had excessive sleepiness (Epworth Sleepiness Scale score of 16/24) and early morning headache as his main symptoms. The patient was taking riluzole (a glutamate antagonist as treatment for his amyotrophic lateral sclerosis) as his only medication. His BMI was 19.8 kg/m^2. Awake arterial blood gas breathing room air was the following: pH 7.40, Paco$_2$ 44 mmHg, and Pao$_2$ 86 mmHg.

A representative 2 minute tracing of REM sleep from his overnight PSG is shown.

An arterial blood gas breathing room air immediately following the overnight PSG showed pH 7.35, Paco$_2$ 52 mmHg, and Pao$_2$ 77 mmHg.

Based on this history, what is the best interpretation of the event depicted in this tracing?

A. An obstructive apnea
B. A central apnea caused by the medication
C. A central hypopnea caused by Cheyne–Stokes breathing
D. Sleep-related hypoventilation
E. Hypopnea from muscle weakness.

Answer on page 203.

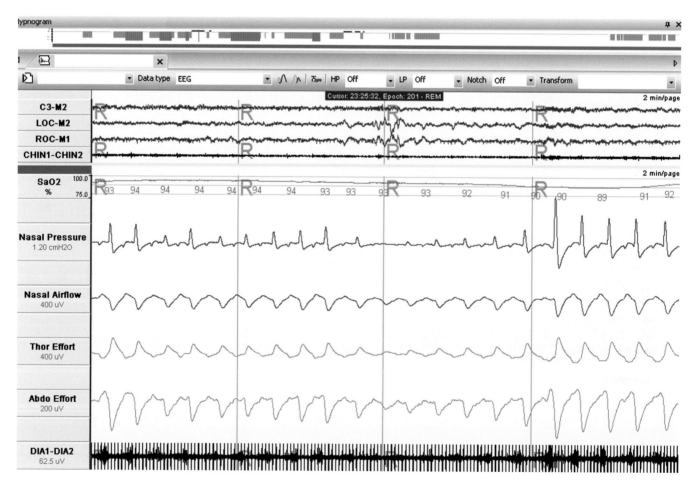

DIA1-DIA2, costal margin surface diaphragmatic EMG; Nasal Airflow, nasal airflow measured by thermistor; Nasal Pressure, nasal airflow measured by nasal pressure transducer; R, REM sleep epoch; Thor Effort, thoracic respiratory inductance plethysmography; Sao$_2$ from finger pulse oximetry.

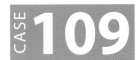
A 54-year-old smoker with chronic obstructive lung disease and a history of snoring, waking up gasping for air, excessive daytime sleepiness, and early morning headaches

Peter J.-C. Wu and John R. Wheatley

A 54-year-old man with a 35 pack-year history of smoking and mild COPD (forced expiratory volume in 1 second [FEV_1] of 3.07 L, or 90% of predicted) presents with polycythemia. Transthoracic echocardiogram showed normal left ventricular function and mild pulmonary hypertension (estimated systolic pulmonary artery pressure of 41 mmHg). The patient gave a history of snoring, waking up gasping for air, excessive daytime sleepiness (Epworth Sleepiness Scale score of 18/24), and early morning headaches. His regular medications included a nicotine patch, bisoprolol, and aspirin; he did not take any sedative medications, narcotics or antihistamines. His BMI was normal, at 23.4 kg/m². On examination, he had no evidence of thoracoabdominal paradox. There were no abnormal findings on examination of his cranial nerves, upper limbs, or lower limbs to suggest a neuropathy or myopathy.

His awake supine arterial blood gas breathing room air demonstrated pH 7.39, $Paco_2$ 49 mmHg, and Pao_2 68 mmHg. A representative 5 minute tracing from his overnight diagnostic PSG is shown in Fig. 1.

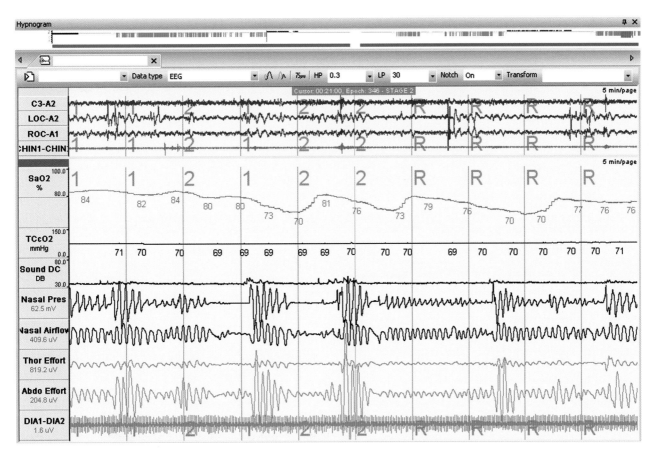

Fig. 1. 1, N1 NREM sleep; 2, N2 NREM sleep; DIA1-DIA2, costal margin surface diaphragmatic EMG; Nasal Airflow, nasal airflow measured by thermistor; Nasal Pres, nasal airflow measured by nasal pressure transducer; R, REM sleep; Sound DC, sound channel recording sound envelope (Db); Thor Effort, thoracic respiratory inductance plethysmography; Sao₂ from finger pulse oximetry.

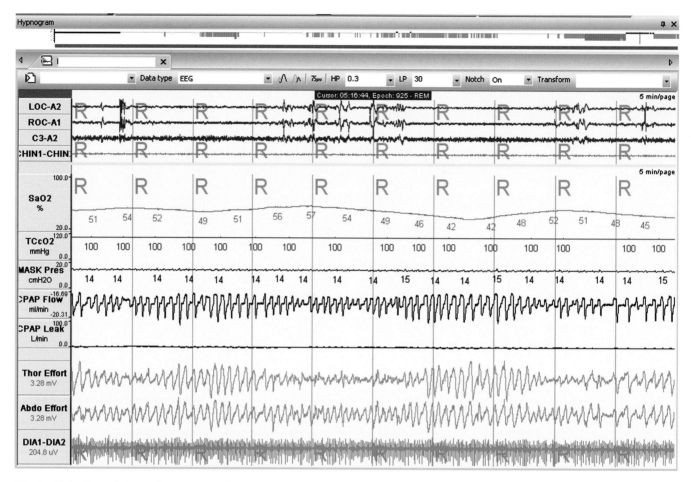

Fig. 2. Abdo Effort, abdominal respiratory inductance plethysmography; CPAP flow, pressure (cmH$_2$O) measured at the mask; CPAP Leak, derived signal indicating unintentional leak from the CPAP system (L/min); DIA1-DIA2, costal margin surface diaphragmatic EMG; MASK Pres, CPAP pressure (cmH$_2$O) measured in the mask; R, REM sleep; Thor Effort, thoracic respiratory inductance plethysmography; SaO2, Spo$_2$ by finger pulse oximetry. Note that the SaO2 and TCcO2 channels are reversed in this tracing.

An arterial blood gas breathing room air on the morning following the overnight PSG demonstrated a pH 7.35, Paco$_2$ 52 mmHg, and Pao$_2$ 65 mmHg.

1. What is the most likely ICSD diagnosis based on the above history and interpretation of the respiratory events displayed on the PSG tracing?

A. Obstructive sleep apnea
B. Central sleep apnea caused by his medications
C. Central sleep apnea as a result of Cheyne–Stokes breathing
D. Idiopathic sleep-related non-obstructive alveolar hypoventilation
E. Obesity-hypoventilation syndrome.

The patient agreed to a trial of CPAP therapy as treatment for a diagnosis of OSA, and initially went on to have a CPAP titration PSG study. No additional treatment or medications were commenced in the interim. The patient was clinically stable at the time of the CPAP titration PSG study. An arterial blood gas sample prior to the study demonstrated pH 7.32, Paco$_2$ 67mmHg, and Pao$_2$ 69mmHg.

Figure 2 shows a representative tracing covering 5 minutes of his CPAP titration study during REM sleep. Figure 3 gives the overnight summary of the CPAP titration study.

An arterial blood gas breathing room air on the morning following the overnight CPAP study had a pH 7.34, Paco$_2$ 62mmHg, and Pao$_2$ 65mmHg.

2. Based on interpretation of these data, what is the best next management step for this patient?

A. Commence patient on nocturnal CPAP therapy
B. Commence patient on nocturnal bilevel PAP in spontaneous mode
C. Commence patient on nocturnal bilevel PAP in spontaneous timed mode
D. Perform an MRI of the brain and brainstem
E. Perform hypoxic and hypercapneic ventilatory responses and test for a mutation of PHOX-2B.

Answer on page 204.

Sex: Male
Weight: 68.5 kg
BMI: 23.4 kg/m2

Height: 171 cm

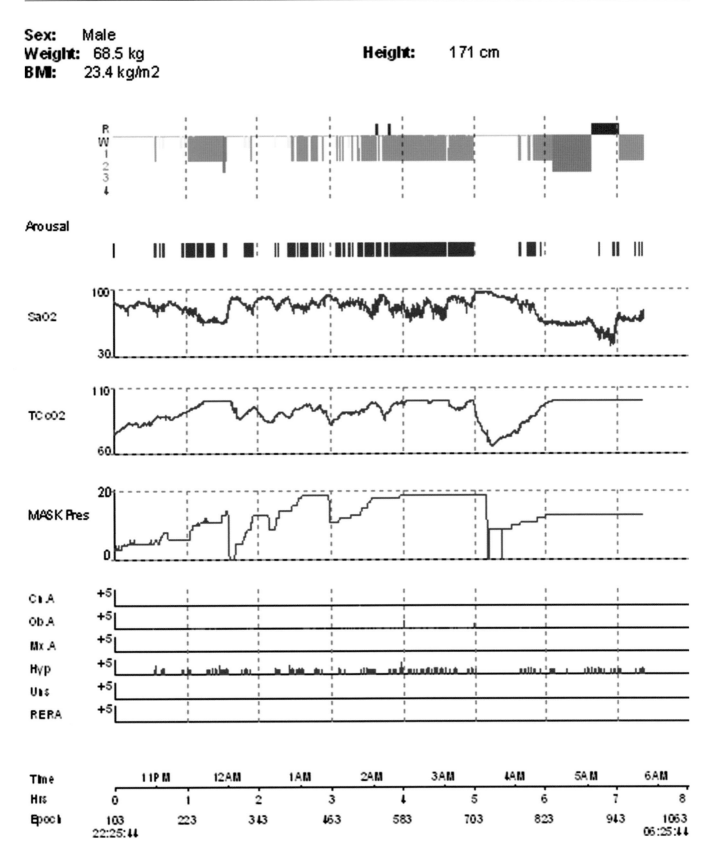

Fig. 3. Arousal, events resulting in EEG arousal; Cn. A, central apnoea; Hyp, hypopnea; MASK Pres, CPAP pressure (cmH$_2$O) measured at the mask; Mx. A, mixed apnea; Ob. A, obstructive apnea; Uns, unsure; SaO2, Spo$_2$ by pulse oximetry.

CASE 110

A 71-year-old woman with a 10 year history of severe obstructive sleep apnea and obesity-hypoventilation syndrome, now with increased daytime sleepiness

Peter J.-C. Wu and John R. Wheatley

A 71-year-old woman was referred to the sleep clinic for re-assessment of sleepiness. She had been diagnosed with severe OSA and obesity-hypoventilation syndrome 10 years previously and had been treated with CPAP at a pressure of 9 cmH$_2$O using a nasal mask since then. She has been diagnosed with multiple comorbidities, including ischemic heart disease, atrial fibrillation, hypertension, congestive cardiac failure, COPD, type 2 diabetes mellitus, and morbid obesity. Over the previous 6 months, she had noticed increased daytime sleepiness, disturbed nocturnal sleep, a dry mouth at night, and decreased exercise tolerance. Her Epworth

Sleepiness Scale was elevated at 13/24. She weighed 96 kg with a BMI of 35.3 kg/m^2, with no significant weight gain over the past 2 years. Her pulse demonstrated atrial fibrillation controlled at a rate of 65 bpm, and blood pressure was normal at 127/73 mmHg. The remainder of her physical examination was unremarkable. Review of her CPAP equipment demonstrated that her mask and tubing were in good condition, sealing well, and her machine pressure was appropriately set at 9 cmH$_2$O. A download of her CPAP machine demonstrated excellent CPAP usage, with an average nightly usage of more than 10 hours. In view of her

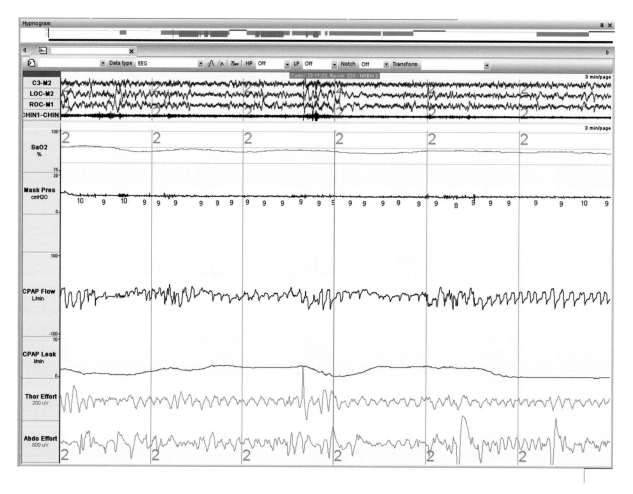

2, NREM stage 2 sleep epoch; Abdo Effort, abdominal respiratory inductance plethysmography; CPAP flow, nasal airflow measured by the CPAP system (L/min); CPAP Leak, derived signal indicating unintentional leak from the CPAP system (L/min); Mask Pres, pressure (cmH$_2$O) measured at the mask; Thor Effort, thoracic respiratory inductance plethysmography; SaO2, Spo$_2$ by pulse oximetry.

continued sleepiness, a CPAP PSG review study was organized to reassess her CPAP pressure.

A representative 3 minute tracing from NREM sleep during the first hour of her overnight PSG is shown.

What is the best interpretation of the respiratory events depicted in this tracing?

A. Obstructive hypopneas resulting from inadequate CPAP machine pressure level

B. Obstructive hypopneas caused by a mask leak

C. A period of Cheyne–Stokes breathing

D. Sleep-related hypoventilation

E. Obstructive hypopneas caused by a mouth air leak.

Answer on page 205.

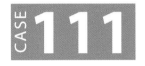

A 20-year-old man with morning headache, excessive daytime sleepiness, heavy snoring, and apnea during sleep

Motoo Yamauchi and Kingman Strohl

A 20-year-old man was referred to the sleep clinic because of the occurrence of morning headache, excessive daytime sleepiness (Epworth Sleepiness Scale score 16/24), and witnessed heavy snoring and apnea during sleep. He had no other significant medical history, including no history of stroke, hypertension, diabetes, or other cardiovascular diseases. In the diagnostic PSG, his AHI was 34.8/h. He was given a tonsillectomy, rather than CPAP, because he is not obese (BMI 24.0 kg/m^2) and he had extremely enlarged tonsils. A 5 minute tracing from the follow-up PSG after tonsillectomy (with the AHI decreased to 4.5/h) is shown.

What is the best interpretation of the respiratory status of this patient as displayed on this tracing?

A. Cheyne–Stokes breathing

B. Central apnea

C. Obstructive apnea under CPAP with optimal pressure

D. Post-sigh pause and sigh-induced Cheyne–Stokes-like breathing

E. Post-sigh normal breathing.

Answer on page 207.

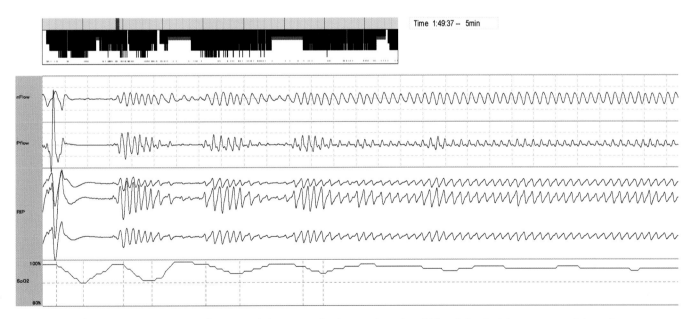

nFlow, thermal sensor; RIP, respiratory inductance plethysmography (upper, thoracic; middle, abdominal; bottom, sum of thoracic and abdominal amplitude).

Case answers

CASE 1

Correct answer: E.

Discussion

A. **Incorrect**. While the history and the changing respiratory pattern suggests this as a possible interpretation, the pattern is irregular rather than "crescendo–decrescendo" for three consecutive cycles, as noted in the American Academy of Sleep Medicine (AASM) Manual as criteria for Cheyne–Stokes breathing.[1] Note that Cheyne–Stokes breathing is less likely associated with REM sleep, the sleep stage depicted here, than non-REM (NREM) sleep.[2]

B. **Incorrect**. The $ETco_2$ shown here does not go above 42 mmHg, which is within normal limits and, therefore, not compatible with hypoventilation in sleep. Further, the Spo_2 never falls below 97%, and without hypoxemia a diagnosis of hypoventilation in a patient breathing room air is not tenable. Finally, the $ETco_2$ is not at least 10 mmHg above the awake Pco_2 value, as necessary to score sleep-related hypoventilation.[1]

C. **Incorrect**. Since there is irregular breathing, as expected in REM sleep as depicted here, no baseline is established from which there is a clear decrease in airflow, particularly not a 50% drop in the thermistor signal, which would be necessary by AASM criteria to score as hypopnea here, given the lack of significant Spo_2 decreases.[1] Further, since there is no significant Spo_2 decrease, hypopnea would be scored only in association with an arousal following the event, and arousals are not clearly scored in this REM period.

D. **Incorrect**. As above for C., there are no clear REM sleep arousals seen, which would necessitate chin EMG as well as EEG change in REM.[1] There is also no evidence of increasing respiratory effort against upper airway resistance, such as flattening of the pressure transducer signal or increasing respiratory effort to score RERAs.[1]

E. **Correct**. There is no respiratory abnormality, and the irregularly irregular breathing without arousal or significant decrease in Spo_2 or increase in $ETco_2$ displayed is normal for REM sleep even in a healthy subject.

REFERENCES

1. Iber C, Ancoli-Israel S, Chesson A for the American Academy of Sleep Medicine. *The AASM Manual for the Scoring of Sleep and Associated Events: Rules, Terminology, and Technical Specifications.* Westchester, IL: American Academy of Sleep Medicine, 2007.

2. Padeletti M, Mooney AM, Green P, Basner RC, Mancini DM. Sleep disordered breathing in patients with acutely decompensated heart failure. *Sleep Med* 2009;**10**:353–360.

CASE 2

Correct answer: D.

Discussion

A. **Incorrect**. While this seems a plausible explanation at first, note that the respiratory rate prior to the "EVENT" is 40/min, not consistent with the stated back-up rate.

B. **Incorrect**. There is no evidence for this; Spo_2 remains the same or is even lower after the "EVENT" point.

C. **Incorrect**. It is true that this is suggested by the better respiratory effort signal that follows from the "EVENT" point; however, such a change by the technologist would likely be accompanied by artifact of such movements. Further, it does not explain the respiratory rate of 40 breaths/min preceding that point nor the immediate change in rate after it. Most likely, the improved respiratory effort signal reflects the fact that the patient is better synchronized with the non-invasive ventilation after the trigger sensitivity change (see D below).

D. **Correct**. The prior signal likely reflects auto-cycling of the non-invasive ventilation, with complete patient–ventilator asynchrony, associated with a trigger sensitivity that was too high (i.e. too sensitive) for the situation, and allowed the machine to auto-cycle rather than respond to the patient's efforts. Once the sensitivity was lowered (made less sensitive), it was able to respond to the patient's respiratory efforts, and generally one-to-one patient–ventilator synchrony is established over the remainder of the epoch displayed. Note, however, that in such a situation lowering the sensitivity may have the effect of promoting patient–ventilator asynchrony by making it too difficult for the patient to trigger the ventilator to assist the effort, particularly in the case of neuromuscular weakness as here. In fact, note that in this tracing, there is evidence of initial respiratory effort by the patient after the trigger sensitivity was decreased, seen most clearly in the abdominal tracing, which is unrewarded by a ventilator assist, with the assist (pressure signal) firing only later with a second inspiratory effort (i.e. ineffective triggering).

E. **Incorrect**. The signal continues to be clearly a bilevel signal of IPAP of 10 cmH$_2$O and EPAP of 4 cmH$_2$O.

FURTHER READING
Suggested reading for patient–ventilator asynchrony with non-invasive ventilation in patients with amyotrophic lateral sclerosis.

Atkeson AD, RoyChoudhury A, Harrington-Moroney G, et al. Patient–ventilator asynchrony with nocturnal non-invasive ventilation in ALS. *Neurology* 2011;**77**:549–555.

CASE 3

Correct answer: B.

Discussion

A. **Incorrect**. The event shows just over 20 seconds of virtually absent respiratory effort: therefore, it is a central apnea. The pressure tracing ("CPRESS") is not a continuous pressure, but a variable bilevel tracing with IPAP set at 4 cmH$_2$O, with slight variation seen breath to breath in this level, and IPAP varying from as high as 17.4 cmH$_2$O during the event, and as low as 6–7 cmH$_2$O seen at the beginning and the end of the tracing. Therefore, this is a non-fixed bilevel PAP mode (see B below).

B. **Correct**. The patient demonstrated Cheyne–Stokes breathing with central sleep apnea at baseline, and this is a central apnea during the use of servo bilevel PAP via a nasal mask. Note that the servo ventilator is supplying a higher inspiratory pressure when the patient's efforts are at a minimum, and a lower inspiratory pressure when the patient's efforts are maximal (before and after the central apnea). There is failure of the servo ventilation to provide ventilation to the patient during this event (the high pressure levels are not transmitted to the chest wall or abdomen; consequently, the patient at this point has neither regularized his breathing efforts nor is receiving ventilatory assistance during his central apnea, two of the expected salutory effects of servo ventilation in patients with Cheyne–Stokes breathing). The reason for this failure is not clear, but may be because of an air leak from the nasal interface, which is interrupting the ventilator's ability to sense effort and/or to deliver pressure to the patient's airway: note the snoring tracing, which may be picking up respiratory signal from the ventilator assists and may represent the airway sounds from this.

C. **Incorrect**. This is central apnea by definition, as per A above. One may look at the snore channel tracing and conclude that there was snoring and, therefore, there is partial airflow with increased resistance, thus potentially hypopnea. But the lack of respiratory effort is incompatible with an interpretation of hypopnea, and likely the snore channel represents another respiratory sound, such as from the inspiratory airflow being delivered to the mask by the servo ventilator.

D. **Incorrect**. As above, this event is central apnea, not hypopnea, and the pressure, while bilevel, is variable rather than fixed: with fixed, the IPAP would be set at one pressure and one pressure would be depicted for each breath, although if there were air leak such a fixed pressure could vary somewhat (i.e. lower than the set pressure).

E. **Incorrect**. There is a correct answer, and that is B.

Follow-up
After adjustment of the interface by the technologist, and decrease in air leak, there was good efficacy of the servo ventilation with amelioration of the Cheyne–Stokes breathing with central apnea, as seen in the PSG tracing which follows. Note that periodic leg movements are now seen.

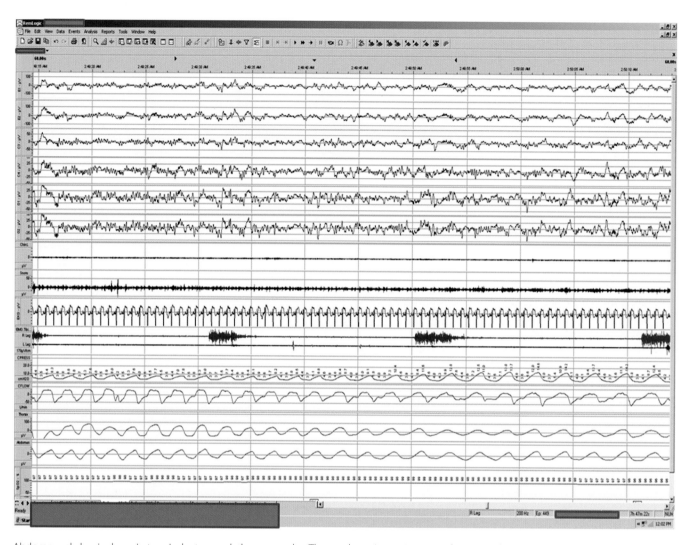

Abdomen, abdominal respiratory inductance plethysmography; Thorax, thoracic respiratory inductance plethysmography; Spo₂ by ear pulse oximetry. Spo₂ displayed remains above 95% throughout the tracing. CPRESS (5th channel from bottom), signal from PAP; EMG tib (6th channel from bottom), right (upper) and left (lower) leg EMG.

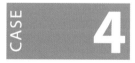

Correct answer: E.

Discussion

A. **Incorrect**. Although this seems plausible at first look (wide biphasic morphology on a right-sided precordial ECG lead), note that the rate is 26; if this is a true signal, it would represent a severe bradycardia rather than normal sinus rhythm.

B. **Incorrect**. If this were a true signal, this is severe bradycardia rather than tachycardia, as noted above.

C. **Incorrect**. One could imagine the small deflections preceding each QRS as flutter waves, but such a slow rate would be incompatible with atrial flutter with 2:1 conduction.[1]

Further, there is good evidence that this ECG signal is artifact (see E below).

D. **Incorrect**. This seems a plausible explanation at first: one could expect a slow wide complex rhythm without clear atrial activity and depression of the ST segment with severe hyperkalemia.[1] However, this is unlikely given the rate, which matches the respiratory rate here, making artifact much more likely. Of note, the patient's potassium levels were checked the next day and were normal.

E. **Correct**. Although this appears to be stage N3 sleep, there appears to be very slow, non-physiologic artifact in the EEG for the first half of the epoch (note the much wider signal up to 1:07:30 a.m.). The ECG displayed is not at the rate of the EEG artifact, however, but is rather at the respiratory rate of 26 breaths/min. This is, therefore, most compatible with respiratory artifact, itself likely promoted by sweating and poor impedance of the ECG channel allowing for this artifact. In fact, subsequent drying of

the chest and replacing the ECG leads immediately resolved this artifact.

REFERENCE

1. Marriot HLJ. *Practical Electrocardiography*, 7th edn. Philadelphia, PA: Williams & Wilkins, 1983.

Correct answer: A.

A. **Correct.** The rhythm is atrial fibrillation. The differential for the wide complex beat that occurs just after 1:43:52 is aberrant ventricular depolarization of a supraventricular beat, or an ectopic ventricular beat. The Ashman phenomenon describes the physiologic fact that an irregular rhythm with variable heart rate is likely to produce aberrant conduction of supraventricular beats, particularly in atrial fibrillation, when a beat ending a short R-R interval following a relatively long R-R interval is likely to be aberrantly conducted.[1,2] Such a setting is true of the wide complex beat here. However, Marriott pointed out in his classic text[2] that such a setting is also conducive to the occurrence of ectopic ventricular beats; consequently, Ashman's phenomenon alone cannot be relied on to determine whether such wide complex beats are, in fact, ventricular ectopic beats or aberrantly conducted beats in the setting of atrial fibrillation.[2]

B. **Incorrect.** There is no evidence of well-defined P waves to interpret this ECG as any type of a "sinus" rhythm.

C. **Incorrect.** While the absence of P waves is compatible with such a diagnosis, the irregularly irregular nature of

the rhythm is not typical of a junctional rhythm,[3] and is classic for atrial fibrillation.

D. **Incorrect.** The rhythm does not have a clear P wave, which would have to be consistently followed by a normal QRS at an increased PR interval (beginning of P wave to beginning of QRS complex $\geqslant 0.21$ seconds)[2] to meet criteria for such a diagnosis.

E. **Incorrect.** As above, although such an ECG could be irregularly irregular, sinus rhythm is not established by a clear P wave with consistent association with a QRS complex, so that sinus rhythm with frequent premature supraventricular beats cannot be interpreted in this tracing.

REFERENCES

1. Gouaux JL, Ashman R. Auricular fibrillation with aberration simulating ventricular paroxysmal tachycardia. *American Heart Journal* 1947;**34**:366.

2. Marriot HLJ. *Practical Electrocardiography*, 7th edn. Philadelphia, PA: Williams & Wilkins, 1983.

3. Mudge GH Jr. *Manual of Electrocardiography*. Boston, MA: Little, Brown, 1981.

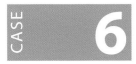

Correct answer: B.

Discussion

A. **Incorrect.** Although snoring is present, as displayed by the snoring channel, such a diagnosis is not part of the AASM Manual for any adult respiratory event,[1] nor would a diagnosis of snoring, which is the most current diagnostic term (previously called "primary snoring") given in the AASM *International Classification of Sleep Disorders* (ICSD),[2] be tenable in this setting, given the consistent hypoxemia. Note that the timing of the snore signal is sometimes inspiratory and sometimes expiratory.

B. **Correct.** This is one of the seven adult PSG respiratory diagnoses outlined in the AASM Manual:[1] the others being the three apneas (central, obstructive, and mixed), hypopnea, Cheyne–Stokes breathing, and RERA. Hypoventilation is diagnosed here by the ET_{CO_2} signal, which reaches 54 mmHg, more than 10 mmHg higher than her awake P_{CO_2}, and is reflected in the consistent hypoxemia displayed throughout the epoch (nadir S_{PO_2} 83%). Note, however, that the degree of hypoxemia appears out of proportion to the level of ET_{CO_2} increase, suggesting a concomitant disorder of gas exchange. Alternatively a disturbance

141

in acid–base status with shift of the oxyhemoglobin dissociation curve to the right, in addition to the hypoventilation, could be contributing to the low O_2 saturation tracing. Note as well that hypoxemia alone is not sufficient to score hypoventilation during sleep as per AASM scoring rules.[1]

C. **Incorrect.** There are no clear arousals (neither EEG nor EMG, the latter necessary to score arousal in REM sleep) associated with any discrete respiratory event such as flattening of the nasal pressure signal or increasing respiratory effort. Further, such an interpretation is not compatible with the consistent hypoxemia and hypercapnia.[1]

D. **Incorrect.** This is REM sleep and there is hypoxemia, but no such classification is currently part of the AASM scoring rules.[1] Further, diagnostic criteria for hypoventilation are met here.

E. **Incorrect.** There is no apnea displayed, nor is such an interpretation present in the AASM scoring rules.[1] Further, such an interpretation would be considered only in the setting of central apneas occurring during CPAP titration, which are not occurring here.[3]

REFERENCES

1. Iber C, Ancoli-Israel S, Chesson A for the American Academy of Sleep Medicine. *The AASM Manual for the Scoring of Sleep and Associated Events: Rules, Terminology, and Technical Specifications.* Westchester, IL: American Academy of Sleep Medicine, 2007.

2. American Academy of Sleep Medicine. *International Classification of Sleep Disorders, Diagnostic and Coding Manual*, 2nd edn. Westchester, IL: American Academy of Sleep Medicine, 2005.

3. Morgenthaler TI, Kagramanov V, Hanak V, *et al.* Complex sleep apnea syndrome: is it a unique clinical syndrome? *Sleep* 2006;**29**:1203.

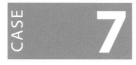

Correct answer: D.

Discussion

A. **Incorrect.** There is no evidence of high $ETco_2$ to diagnose hypoventilation nor to explain the consistent hypoxemia;[1] in fact, the $ETco_2$ tracing is registering in the low 20 mmHg range, likely artifactually low.

B. **Incorrect.** There is no apnea.

C. **Incorrect.** Snoring is present on the snore channel, although it is not clear how true this signal is given that the snore signal varies between inspiration and expiration. However, snoring alone cannot be diagnosed in the presence of hypoxemia.

D. **Correct.** There is no evidence of apnea, hypopnea, or hypoventilation to explain this hypoxemia.[1] Most importantly, note the heart rate being registered by the pulse oximeter in the bottom-most channel on this tracing: very slow, and nowhere in the range of the true heart rate seen in the ECG (73 bpm over this epoch). Therefore, the inference is that the pulse oximeter is not adequately picking up the pulse signal here, either for accurate heart rate or Spo_2 measurement. Further evidence for artifact is seen at the very end of the tracing, where the last two channels show a complete loss of the oximeter signal for both Spo_2 and heart rate, suggesting that the oximeter was not attached adequately prior to this.

E. **Incorrect.** Such a diagnosis is made when central apneas are present during initial titration of CPAP for OSA;[2] there are no central apneas here, nor is CPAP being used.

REFERENCES

1. Iber C, Ancoli-Israel S, Chesson A for the American Academy of Sleep Medicine. *The AASM Manual for the Scoring of Sleep and Associated Events: Rules, Terminology, and Technical Specifications.* Westchester, IL: American Academy of Sleep Medicine, 2007.

2. Gay PC. Complex sleep apnea: it really is a disease. *J Clin Sleep Med* 2008;**4**:403–405.

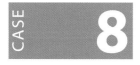

Correct answer: F.

Discussion

A, B, and C. **Incorrect.** Each of these findings is present here. However, *all* of these must be present in an epoch to score it as stage R.[1]

D. **Incorrect.** Sawtooth waves are present here, characteristically maximal in the central derivations and just preceding a burst of eye movements. However, such activity is neither necessary nor sufficient for scoring an epoch as stage R and is not, in fact, in the current scoring rules as a criterion for scoring stage R.[1]

E. **Incorrect**. Irregular shallow airflow and breathing efforts are present, particularly between 4:41:05 and 4:41:15 a.m. Such breathing is characteristic of REM but is neither necessary nor sufficient to score an epoch as stage R sleep, and is not, in fact, in the current scoring rules as a criterion for scoring stage R.[1]

F. **Correct**. None of the above answers are correct. See A above.

REFERENCE

1. Iber C, Ancoli-Israel S, Chesson A for the American Academy of Sleep Medicine. *The AASM Manual for the Scoring of Sleep and Associated Events: Rules, Terminology, and Technical Specifications.* Westchester, IL: American Academy of Sleep Medicine, 2007.

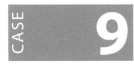

Correct answer: F.

Discussion

A. **Incorrect**. The event can indeed be considered to fulfill AASM scoring rules for an obstructive apnea,[1] *if* one judges that the "peak thermal sensor" excursion displayed here represents a fall of at least 90% from baseline, which appears possible from this tracing. Note that the nasal pressure transducer signal above the thermistor signal cannot be used to score apnea here, even though it appears flat (e.g. the patient may be mouth breathing). Note as well that the current rules, while stated to imply a quantitative criterion, really leave the interpreter to make a qualitative decision, for example at what point of the "baseline" is the drop in the sensor to be measured? How and where is "baseline" quantified? How can 90% (apnea) versus 89% (hypopnea) be quantified here (particularly from a non-calibrated thermal sensor signal)? Consequently, while obstructive apnea may be judged to be correct, other possibilities also appear correct (see below) such that "obstructive apnea only" is not the most accurate response here.

B. **Incorrect**. Hypopnea can indeed be scored here *if* the interpreter judges that the peak thermal sensor drop is at least 30% but less than 90% of the baseline (note that the degree of O_2 desaturation [from 97% to 92%] outright fits hypopnea scoring rules if a 30–89% decrease in the flow sensor is also adjudicated). Therefore, while hypopnea may be judged to be present, other possibilities also appear correct (see above and below) such that "hypopnea only" is not the most accurate response here.

C. **Incorrect**. Hypoventilation is technically present according to AASM scoring rules,[1] which state that hypoventilation is scored if there is at least a 10 mmHg increase in the $ETCO_2$ (as a surrogate marker of PCO_2) during sleep compared with an awake baseline value. Note that neither a necessary minimal nor maximal duration of such an event is specified in the AASM *Scoring Manual*. However, while hypoventilation may be scored, other scoring can also be correct (see above and below) such that "hypoventilation only" is not the most accurate response here.

D. **Incorrect**. There is no clear arousal from sleep, and the event meets criteria for either an apnea or a hypopnea as above: both of these rule out RERA as a correct interpretation.

E. **Incorrect**. Even if the event is judged to meet apnea rather than hypopnea criteria (see A and B above), there is no indication of absent respiratory effort in the initial portion of the event to score as mixed apnea.

F. **Correct**. As discussed above, the events stated in A, B, or C are all scoreable here, depending upon a basically subjective decision regarding the degree of airflow decrease. Note that the current AASM scoring rules do not specify how to interpret an event when it fits more than one criterion for scoring, or whether such interpretations are or are not mutually exclusive. In practice, however, it must be recognized that the decision regarding scoring will have important ramifications regarding the apnea hypopnea index (AHI) (hypoventilation alone does not add to the AHI), the overall interpretation of the study (e.g. OSA, or one of the alveolar hypoventilation syndromes),[2] and possibly the treatment applied (e.g. CPAP versus bilevel PAP). As a further complexity here, note that the current ICSD Manual[2] criteria for diagnosing one of the hypoventilation syndromes does not require the $ETCO_2$ increase that is required for scoring a hypoventilation event in sleep in the AASM scoring rules.[1]

REFERENCES

1. Iber C, Ancoli-Israel S, Chesson A for the American Academy of Sleep Medicine. *The AASM Manual for the Scoring of Sleep and Associated Events: Rules, Terminology, and Technical Specifications.* Westchester, IL: American Academy of Sleep Medicine, 2007.

2. American Academy of Sleep Medicine. *International Classification of Sleep Disorders, Diagnostic and Coding Manual*, 2nd edn. Westchester, IL: American Academy of Sleep Medicine, 2005.

Correct answer: B.

Discussion

A. **Incorrect**. The pattern of central apneas here is irregular rather than "waxing/waning" for three consecutive cycles, as would be necessary as criteria for Cheyne–Stokes breathing.[1]

B. **Correct**. Displayed are the servo ventilation (CPRESS) and associated mask airflow (FLOW) channels, giving the default back-up rate ventilator assist at 15/min, with virtually no relationship to the patient's efforts, as displayed on the thoracic and abdominal effort channels. Indeed, at many times there are fairly prolonged central apneas, with the servo device not delivering effective ventilation despite giving the "back-up;" in line with this, note the severe O_2 desaturation following the two longest central apneas, particularly the last, and despite the ventilator firing consistently at the back-up rate of 15/minute.

Air leak was noted by the technologist and is likely to be contributing to this asynchrony between ventilator and patient effort here.

C. **Incorrect**. These are central apneas: mixed apneas begin central but end obstructive.[1]

D. **Incorrect**. As noted for B, this is not the expected response: the expected response is a 1:1 matching of ventilator assist with patient effort, with abolishment of central apnea, and indeed less-apparent periodic breathing when used in this setting of heart failure and Cheyne–Stokes breathing.

E. **Incorrect**, since choice B is correct.

REFERENCE

1. Iber C, Ancoli-Israel S, Chesson A for the American Academy of Sleep Medicine. *The AASM Manual for the Scoring of Sleep and Associated Events: Rules, Terminology, and Technical Specifications.* Westchester, IL: American Academy of Sleep Medicine, 2007.

Correct answer: D.

Discussion

A. **Incorrect**. Sick sinus syndrome is recognized by bursts of atrial tachyarrhythmia followed by periods of sinus node and/or junctional inertia (e.g. marked sinus bradycardia, sinus arrest, or sinoatrial block). No tachycardia or bradycardia occurs here, although there is periodic sinus acceleration and deceleration. The rhythm shown in the first figure does not clearly show P waves, although these are clearly present in the second figure.[1]

B. **Incorrect**. Wolff–Parkinson–White syndrome classically consists of a short PR interval, with a wide QRS complex whose initial deflection is slurred ("delta wave"); associated reciprocating tachyarrhythmias, atrial flutter, or fibrillation, and even ventricular fibrillation, may occur.[1] None of these features is present in the tracing shown.

C. **Incorrect**. There is no evidence of a paced rhythm (e.g. the presence of pacer spikes) in either tracing.

D. **Correct**. This is likely sinus arrhythmia associated with cyclic obstructive apnea and arousal, with slowing particularly evident just prior to the termination of the obstructive event (possibly associated with vagal stimulation from expiratory effort against the closed airway

and/or Hering–Breuer reflex) as well as following the arousal and its associated sinus acceleration (the slowing likely from a baroreflex response). Figure 1A does not clearly demonstrate P waves in this compressed 60 second figure, although clear P waves are seen on the 30 second tracing in Fig. 1B. Although there is heart rate slowing and acceleration, there is no tachycardia (i.e. an average heart rate > 100 bpm) or bradycardia (i.e. average heart rate < 60 bpm) achieved.[1]

Further note

Note that the definitions of bradycardia and tachycardia above.[1] differ from AASM recommendations of scoring sinus tachycardia as sustained sinus heart rate > 90 bpm for adults, and sinus bradycardia as sustained heart rate < 40 bpm for ages 6 years through adult.[2] Note also that the sinus arrhythmia seen here differs from the sinus arrhythmia associated with breathing, in which heart rate accelerates with inspiration and decelerates with expiration,[1] possibly because any such respiratory sinus arrhythmia is superseded by the stimuli of the apneas and arousals here.

The following tracings in Fig. 2 show the same ECGs in the context of the entire PSG, each 60 seconds, illustrating the obstructive apneas and arousals associated with the arrhythmia (A),

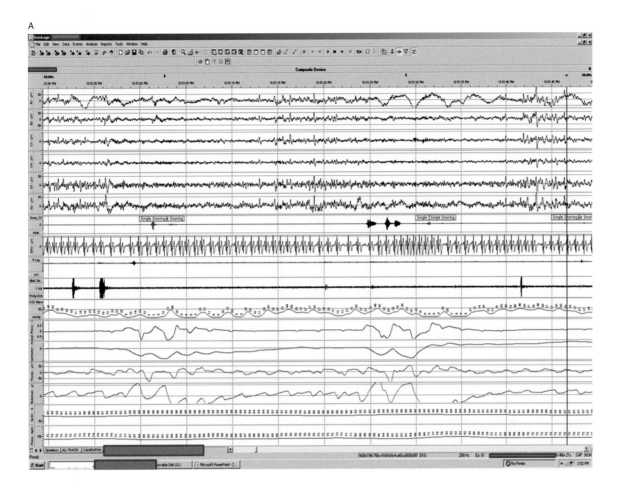

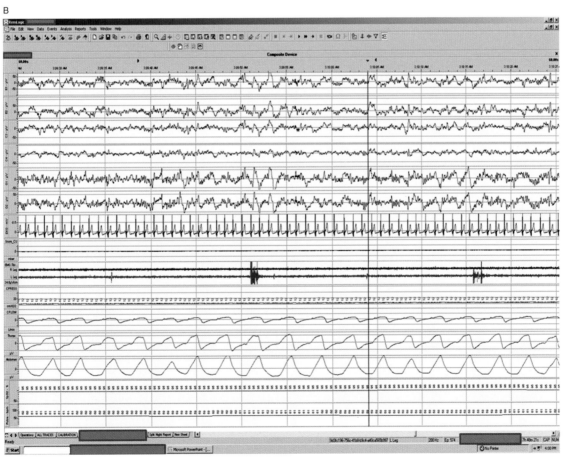

Fig. 2. Abdomen, abdominal respiratory inductance plethysmography; Cc, central referential EEG; Nasal pressure; nasal pressure transducer; Thorax, thoracic respiratory inductance plethysmography; Spo$_2$ from ear pulse oximetry.

followed by the resolution of the arrhythmia, with resolution of the sleep apnea, with the use of CPAP (here set at 12 cmH$_2$O) (B).

REFERENCES

1. Marriot HLJ. *Practical Electrocardiography*, 7th edn. Philadelphia, PA: Williams & Wilkins, 1983.

2. Iber C, Ancoli-Israel S, Chesson A for the American Academy of Sleep Medicine. *The AASM Manual for the Scoring of Sleep and Associated Events: Rules, Terminology, and Technical Specifications.* Westchester, IL: American Academy of Sleep Medicine, 2007.

CASE 12

Question 1

Correct answer: C.

Discussion

A. **Incorrect**. The event is best interpreted as a "mixed" apnea given the lack of inspiratory effort during the first part of the apnea pictured (note that the beginning of the apnea does not appear to be displayed here).[1] The treatment pictured is not CPAP, but bilevel PAP (IPAP is 11–12 cmH$_2$O; EPAP is approximately 6 cmH$_2$O).

B. **Incorrect**. As above, this event is best interpreted as mixed rather than obstructive apnea.[1]

C. **Correct**, as discussed above. Note the severe O$_2$ desaturation associated with this event.

D. **Incorrect**. Hypoventilation cannot be scored by AASM rules given the lack of a Pco$_2$ measurement; note that O$_2$ desaturation alone does not meet criteria for sleep-related hypoventilation.[1] CPAP is not being used, as noted above.

E. **Incorrect**. This is not spontaneous breathing but rather breathing with bilevel PAP. Further, the event is better interpreted as mixed than central apnea since there is clearly obstructed effort for at least two breaths (and likely partial obstruction for another breath prior to resolution of the event) despite the lack of effort on the first part of the apnea as displayed.

Further note regarding "mixed apnea" scoring

The rules set out by the AASM do not specify the length of absent inspiratory effort for the first part of the apnea nor length of the period of "resumption of inspiratory effort" for the second part of the apnea necessary to score the event as mixed apnea.[1] Further, these rules do not specify definitions for scoring apneas and hypopneas during PAP use; in the given tracing, for example, there is no thermal sensor to define an apnea as a "≥ 90% drop in the peak thermal sensor excursion."

Question 2

Correct answer: A.

Discussion

A. **Correct**. There is sinus rhythm, with two non-conducted P waves during the apnea displayed. It is difficult to assess from this lead whether "type 1" or "type 2" block is present. Type 1 (also sometimes referred to as "Wenckebach type," although Wenckebach actually described both type 1 and type 2, prior to Mobitz) is associated classically with progressive lengthening of the PR interval prior to the dropped beat (this is correctly referred to as the "Wenckebach phenomenon"). This is not clearly evident for the non-conducted P waves seen here.[2] However, type 2 AV block is most commonly associated with bilateral bundle branch block, and thus the QRS is usually widened in that setting,[2] although this is not the case here. The block occurring here is likely contributed to by the combined and reversible cholinergic effects of the REM sleep and the vagal influence of the obstructed breathing.

B. **Incorrect**. First-degree AV block is recognized by prolongation of the PR interval, not present here, and does not include dropped beats.[2]

C. **Incorrect**. Third-degree ("complete") AV block is defined by the absence of sinus activity being conducted to the ventricle; therefore, P waves and the QRS complex occur at rates independent of each other. The tracing shows clear association between the P wave and the QRS for the majority of the beats.

D. **Incorrect**. Atrial flutter is not present as there are clear P waves conducted 1:1 to the QRS for most of the tracing, and no activity suggestive of flutter waves.[2] The ECG activity at 2:19:22 is, however, not clear: there is movement at that time and this appears to affect the ECG signal (likely artifact). One or two dropped P waves are possible; an ectopic atrial wave followed by a wide QRS as a result of aberrant conduction is also possible. Atrial fibrillation, if one determined there is no clear P wave activity, is also possible in this period, although this is too short a time to define this, particularly given the likely movement artifact.

REFERENCES

1. Iber C, Ancoli-Israel S, Chesson A for the American Academy of Sleep Medicine. *The AASM Manual for the Scoring of Sleep and Associated Events: Rules, Terminology, and Technical Specifications.* Westchester, IL: American Academy of Sleep Medicine, 2007.

2. Marriot HLJ. *Practical Electrocardiography*, 7th edn. Philadelphia, PA: Williams & Wilkins, 1983.

Correct answer: A.

Discussion

A. **Correct**. The event is 30 seconds of absent inspiratory effort throughout the entire period of absent airflow, thus meeting criteria for central apnea. Note that the beginning of the event is not pictured here, but based on current scoring rules,[1] this does not impact on the definition of this event as a central apnea.

B. **Incorrect**. As per A above

C. **Incorrect**. Although central apnea is a characteristic finding in Cheyne–Stokes breathing and the nadir of the decrescendo breathing, the pictured tracing does not show at least three consecutive cycles of crescendo–decrescendo breathing necessary for such scoring.[1]

D. **Incorrect**. The event is not associated with a $Paco_2$ level of at least 10 mmHg compared with the awake supine level (here the $ETco_2$ tracing is used as the $Paco_2$).[1]

E. **Incorrect**. Central apnea is clearly defined and can be scored (but see following tracing and discussion). Note that, when respiratory effort resumes, there is crescendo airflow for approximately 10 seconds. This cannot be reliably scored as hypopnea, as the only "baseline"[1] to compare the excursion of the airflow sensors is a flat line (apnea); consequently, this period cannot be defined as showing a "drop" in the airflow tracing excursion compared with what precedes it.

Further note

The following is a 5 minute PSG tracing that includes the central apnea depicted in the tracing on p. 14.

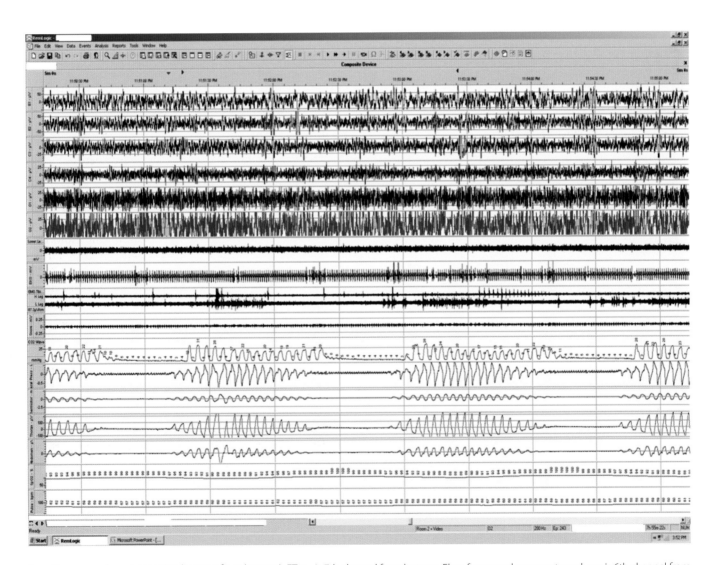

Spo$_2$ from ear pulse oximeter (2nd tracing from bottom). ETco$_2$ is 7th channel from bottom. Flow from nasal pressure transducer is 6th channel from bottom. Oronasal thermistor airflow is 5th channel from bottom. Abdominal and thoracic efforts are 3rd and 4th channels from bottom, respectively.

This tracing now is consistent with an interpretation of Cheyne–Stokes breathing by the AASM scoring rules for respiratory events,[1] although not in itself sufficient to score "central sleep apnea as a result of a Cheyne–Stokes breathing pattern"[2] unless it is determined that there are five or more central apneas or hypopneas per hour of sleep, or that such cyclic crescendo–decrescendo breathing has a duration of at least 10 consecutive minutes.[2] Note that each period of absent inspiratory effort and airflow pictured, including the one discussed above, is scored as a central apnea. Therefore, if there are at least five central apneas per hour within this cyclic breathing, this represents a situation in which two different types of respiratory "event" are scored for the same event (i.e. Cheyne–Stokes breathing; central apnea), although how best to score multiple respiratory abnormalities for the same event is not specifically discussed in the current AASM Manual.[1]

REFERENCES
1. Iber C, Ancoli-Israel S, Chesson A for the American Academy of Sleep Medicine. *The AASM Manual for the Scoring of Sleep and Associated Events: Rules, Terminology, and Technical Specifications.* Westchester, IL: American Academy of Sleep Medicine, 2007.
2. American Academy of Sleep Medicine. *International Classification of Sleep Disorders, Diagnostic and Coding Manual*, 2nd edn. Westchester, IL: American Academy of Sleep Medicine, 2005.

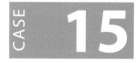

Correct answer: D.

Discussion

A. **Incorrect**. Although there is respiratory-associated variation in the ECG signal, this term refers to changing heart rate rather than changing amplitude; only the latter is apparent here.

B. **Incorrect**. This term in fact denotes an alternating QRS amplitude, often seen with pericardial effusion.[1] However, "alternans" in this setting typically refers to a beat to beat alternation of amplitude, not alternation that varies with respiration and is not beat to beat, as on the current tracing. Also see D below.

C. **Incorrect**. Pulsus alternans (or mechanical alternans) is a clinical rather than an ECG diagnosis, although electrical alternans may be seen when there is pulsus alternans.

D. **Correct**. As noted above, electrical alternans would be associated with a beat to beat alternation in amplitude, which is not the case here. The major indicator of artifact here is that the leg EMG (seen in the channel just below the ECG) is not shifting amplitude with breathing as is the ECG lead, suggesting that the changes in amplitude on the ECG channel are artifactual, and the result of movement of the chest wall with inspiration/expiration rather than a true shift in voltage of the ECG signal.

E. **Incorrect**. This term refers to alternation of the P wave as well as the QRS, and has been described in cardiac tamponade, particularly that related to a malignant pericardial effusion.[1] The current tracing shows a changing of only the QRS, and not the P wave.

REFERENCE
1. Marriot HLJ. *Practical Electrocardiography*, 7th edn. Philadelphia, PA: Williams & Wilkins, 1983.

Correct answer: C.

Discussion

This tracing shows that the patient has a sleep-related breathing disorder, likely OSA. The indicated section is a burst of rhythmic, diffuse spike-wave activity seen in all the displayed EEG channels. It appears during the arousal from a hypopnea, potentially leading to confusion with a movement arousal.

A. **Incorrect**. This entity usually consists of diffuse slowing, often accompanied by EMG artifact. In this example, the EEG change is also seen in the EOG channels – where a REM continues during the discharge, making arousal unlikely.

B. **Incorrect**. Movement artifact would likely be seen in all channels, and also would be unlikely during a REM.

C. **Correct**. This discharge is at a regular 3 Hz frequency, and with careful examination a distinct spike-wave pattern is evident. This pattern can be difficult to see on a limited EEG montage and is often more evident at a slower speed. The patient was taking phenytoin, an anticonvulsant; on further history he had a well-controlled generalized seizure disorder, most likely juvenile myoclonic epilepsy.[1] Generalized tonic–clonic (grand mal) seizures in this syndrome tend to occur mostly during the transition between sleep and wakefulness, and particularly in the early morning. These patients also have myoclonic seizures, consisting of brief jerking of extremities; this also tends to happen on awakening.[2] Absence seizures can be present as well. The characteristic EEG pattern is 3 Hz generalized spike and wave, as seen in this case. Occurrence of OSA is common in the general population; however, it is more common in patients with epilepsy where, untreated, it can contribute to epilepsy intractability.[3]

D. **Incorrect**. This would be present preferentially in the snore channel.

E. **Incorrect**. The posterior dominant rhythm is seen only in posterior EEG electrodes, and has a much faster frequency (8.5–13 Hz) than the indicated pattern.

REFERENCES
1. Dhanuka AK, Jain BK, Daljit S, Maheshiwari D. Juvenile myoclonic epilepsy: a clinical and sleep EEG study. *Seizure* 2001; **10**:374–378.
2. Wolf P, Schmitt JJ. Awakening epilepsies and juvenile myoclonic epilepsy. In *Sleep and Epilepsy: The Clinical Spectrum*, Bazil MB, Malow BA, Sammaritano MR (eds.). Amsterdam: Elsevier, 2002, pp. 237–243.
3. Malow BA, Levy K, Maturen K, Bowes R. Obstructive sleep apnea is common in medically refractory epilepsy patients. *Neurology* 2000; **55**:1002–1007.

CASE 16

Correct answer: B.

Discussion

By history, the patient most likely has narcolepsy. This diagnosis requires excessive daytime somnolence not explained by other sleep disorders. Additional supportive symptoms may be present, including hypnic hallucinations, sleep paralysis, and cataplexy; this patient had all of these. Although each can occur sporadically in the general population, and can sometimes be exacerbated by sleep deprivation from any cause, the clinical history is consistent with narcolepsy with cataplexy.

A PSG study is often performed to rule out other causes of sleep disruption, although PSG followed by a multiple sleep latency test (MSLT) is not required for the diagnosis.

A. **Incorrect**. Excessive daytime somnolence is, in fact, required for a diagnosis of narcolepsy.

B. **Correct**. The age is typical (usual onset is between 15 and 25 years) but the sudden onset is unusual. Often symptoms will be recognized with a change in habits, and in this case may appear abrupt. For example, students with flexible schedules may function quite well with narcolepsy, self-treating with daytime naps. However, once they enter the workforce and are required to be alert for 8 or more consecutive hours on the job, excessive sleepiness may become evident.

C. **Incorrect**. This is cataplexy. Although classically cataplexy occurs with emotion (laughter or fear), startle is not uncommon as a trigger.

D. **Incorrect**. Disturbed nocturnal sleep, as evident in this hypnogram, is frequent in narcolepsy. A PSG study may be necessary to determine whether other conditions, such as OSA, are present and contributing to daytime sleepiness. If so, these must first be treated before evaluation with MSLT.

Note that the displayed hypnogram does not show a sleep-onset REM (SOREM) period, although the REM onset latency is short.

Follow-up

The patient underwent MSLT, which showed a mean sleep latency of 0.3 minutes, and REM sleep in two of four nap opportunities. This was, therefore, supportive of narcolepsy. On further questioning, the patient stated that she had been using cocaine and amphetamines daily since about age 18, and she had recently entered a drug rehabilitation program. She had, therefore, been off stimulants for the past month, likely contributing to the rather sudden recognition of excessive sleepiness in her case.

FURTHER READING
Broughton WA, Broughton RJ. Psychosocial impact of narcolepsy. *Sleep* 1994;**17**(Suppl):S45–S49.
Dauvilliers Y, Tafti M. Molecular genetics and treatment of narcolepsy. *Ann Med* 2006;**38**:252–262.
Morgenthaler TI, Kapur VK, Brown TM, *et al.* Practice parameters for the treatment of narcolepsy and other hypersomnias of central origin. *Sleep* 2007;**30**:1705–1711.

Question 1

Correct answer: D.

Discussion

A. **Incorrect.** PLMs are shown at a frequency of about 25 seconds. However, only one is associated with an electrographic arousal. Assuming that this is typical of his movements on this study, the movements are unlikely to be associated with the insomnia. However, such movements could trigger parasomnias, including sleep-walking and sleep-talking.

B. **Incorrect.** See A.

C. **Incorrect.** See A.

D. **Correct.** See A.

E. **Incorrect.** See A.

Question 2

Correct answer: D.

Discussion

A. **Incorrect.** Although this is a sought-for finding, particularly hearing this history, the displayed EMG does not show the diagnostic criteria as elaborated in the ICSD-2: "excessive amounts of sustained or intermittent elevation of submental EMG tone or excessive phasic submental or (upper or lower) limb EMG twitching."[1] See also D below.

B. **Incorrect.** No obstructive events are depicted.

C. **Incorrect.** No CO_2 data are displayed, nor is the Spo_2 decreased to suggest such a disorder.

D. **Correct.** While excessive EMG activity, as in A above, might have initially been scored, note that the submental EMG is discharging in phase with the ECG, indicating ECG artifact rather than the excessive EMG activity characteristic of REM sleep without atonia.

Follow-up

Given no other significant findings on PSG, and the parasomnia he displayed during the study, he was given a diagnosis of REM sleep behavior disorder (RBD).[2] There were no subsequent findings suggestive of neurodegenerative disease.[3] It is possible that his disorder was exacerbated by chronic insomnia; therefore, clonazepam was recommended, with clinical improvement in the insomnia and parasomnia. Melatonin was also tried but did not result in significant improvement.

REFERENCES

1. American Academy of Sleep Medicine. *International Classification of Sleep Disorders, Diagnostic and Coding Manual,* 2nd edn. Westchester, IL: American Academy of Sleep Medicine, 2005.

2. Gugger JJ, Wagner ML. Rapid eye movement sleep behavior disorder. *Ann Pharmacother* 2007;**41**:1833–1841.

3. Postuma RB, Gagnon JF, Vendette M, *et al.* Quantifying the risk of neurodegenerative disease in idiopathic REM sleep behavior disorder. *Neurology* 2009;**72**:1296–1300.

CASE

18

Correct answer: B.

Discussion

A. **Incorrect.** The tracing shows PLMs of sleep, with a periodicity of about 25 seconds. Most of the movements are associated with an electrographic arousal, making this likely to be clinically relevant, as daytime sleepiness may be seen with PLM disorder.[1]

B. **Correct.** The main symptom is sudden attacks of drowsiness. This is not behavior typical of PLMs but could be related.[1] Appropriate treatments for PLMs of sleep include gabapentinoids (gabapentin enacarbil is the only one that is approved by the US Food and Drug Administration; however, there is some evidence that gabapentin and pregabalin may also be effective).[2,3] Dopamine agonists (ropinirole and pramipexole are approved by the US Food and Drug Administration), benzodiazepines, and opiates may also be considered. Most clinicians feel that gabapentinoids are less effective than dopamine agonists, but these probably have a more favorable adverse effect profile and so are reasonable treatments, particularly in this setting where it is unclear that such treatment will result in improvement of her sleepiness.

C. **Incorrect.** The findings are possibly relevant (see response to B); however, eszopiclone is not an appropriate treatment for this condition. It is indicated for insomnia only and is more appropriate for sleep-maintenance insomnia given the relatively long half-life (6 hours).

D. **Incorrect.** Although PLMs of sleep could be contributing to drowsiness, the symptoms described are unusually severe; therefore, it is by no means certain that this is the only problem. The patient should be assessed for other conditions, including other sleep disorders (such as narcolepsy) and other conditions of hypersomnia causing sudden loss of awareness, particularly syncope and epilepsy.[4]

E. **Incorrect.** For reasons noted above.

REFERENCES

1. American Academy of Sleep Medicine. *International Classification of Sleep Disorders, Diagnostic and Coding Manual,* 2nd edn. Westchester, IL: American Academy of Sleep Medicine, 2005.

2. Garcia-Borreguero D, Larrosa O, de la Llave Y, *et al.* Treatment of restless legs syndrome with gabapentin: a double-blind, cross-over study. *Neurology* 2002;**59**:1573–1579.

3. Allen R, Chen C, Soaita A, *et al.* A randomized, double-blind, 6-week, dose-ranging study of pregabalin in patients with restless legs syndrome. *Sleep Med* 2010;**11**:512–519.

4. Natarajan R. Review of periodic limb movement and restless leg syndrome. *J Postgrad Med* 2010;**56**:157.

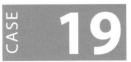

CASE 19

Correct answer: E.

Discussion

A. **Incorrect.** Although bursts of rhythmic activity can occur with arousal, these are usually limited or absent after childhood. They are also typically delta frequency ($< 4\,Hz$); the indicated discharge is much faster.

B. **Incorrect.** Movement artifact would be much more irregular, and would typically be seen on non-cerebral channels as well (such as the ECG).

C. **Incorrect.** Lambda waves are rhythmic sharp waves seen with scanning vision, such as looking at a pattern on the wall or reading. This would not occur directly from sleep.

D. **Incorrect.** The indicated discharge is diffuse rather than posterior, and more prominent anteriorly.

E. **Correct.** Although difficult to fully appreciate the rhythmic activity with the limited sleep-staging PSG montage, as shown in Fig.1, the description of sudden awakening with chaotic movements is entirely consistent with nocturnal frontal lobe epilepsy.[1] Such patients may have several

episodes per night, although some have them more sporadically or rarely. Epileptic seizures rarely arise from REM sleep and, therefore, tend to occur earlier rather than later in a night's sleep.[2] Strictly speaking, nocturnal frontal lobe epilepsy only occurs during sleep; however, other frontal lobe seizures can begin while the patient is awake, usually making distinction from parasomnias easier in that regard.[3] Seizures can also occur in clusters. The characteristic activity is optimally seen in the full-montage EEG in Fig. 2.

REFERENCES

1. Derry CP. The sleep manifestations of frontal lobe epilepsy. *Curr Neurol Neurosci Rep* 2011;**11**:218–226.

2. Herman ST, Walczak TS, Bazil CW. Distribution of partial seizures during the sleep–wake cycle: differences by seizure onset site. *Neurology* 2001;**56**:1453–1459.

3. Zucconi M, Ferini-Strambi L. NREM parasomnias: arousal disorders and differentiation from nocturnal frontal lobe epilepsy. *Clin Neurophysiol* 2000;**111**(Suppl 2):S129–S135.

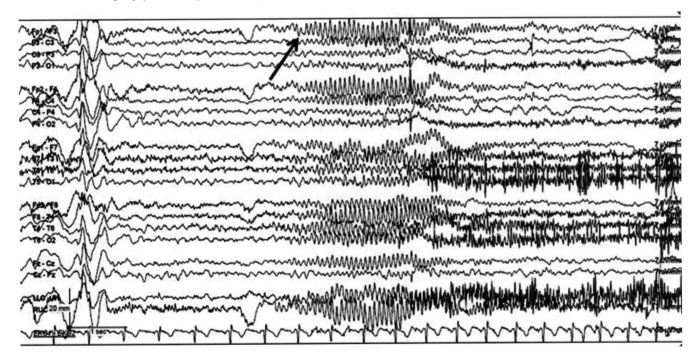

Fig. 2.

Correct answer: E.

Discussion

The tracing shows a regular rhythm, but indistinct P waves and a poorly defined baseline. The following tracing helps to clarify the scoring.

This is the same tracing but using a modified lead II. Note the improved clarity of the P wave with the use of lead II, whose vector traverses the atria. Sinus rhythm with clear P waves conducted to the QRS is now apparent. Without such clarification, atrial fibrillation could be considered with the wavering baseline without clear P waves, and the history of

paroxysmal atrial fibrillation, although the regularity of the rhythm argues against such a diagnosis.

A. **Incorrect**. The lead I tracing has a lack of clear P waves and an indistinct baseline, which do not allow for a scoring of sinus rhythm despite the regularity of the rhythm.
B. **Incorrect**. As noted above.
C. **Incorrect**. Tachycardia is not present with the noted rate of 80 bpm.
D. **Incorrect**. Primarily for the same reason as above.
E. **Correct**. As noted above.

Modified Lead II

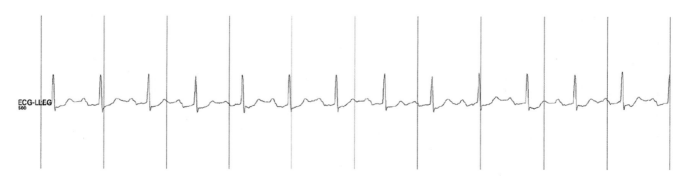

ECG-LLEG
500

Correct answer: D.

Discussion

A–C. **Incorrect**. This is a paced rhythm, with pacer spikes seen before each myocardial discharge.
D. **Correct**. Note that there is also present a paroxysmal run of wide complex beats at a rate >100 bpm. The single ECG channel is limited by the inability to determine the origin

of a widened QRS complex (ventricular versus supraventricular), although the lack of conduction from the atrium (note the pacer spike seen prior to the third wide complex beat) suggests that these are of ventricular origin. Therefore, the best answer is "none of the above" for the underlying rhythm, and the best interpretation from this tracing is "wide complex tachycardia," the origin of which cannot be determined.

Correct answer: B.

Discussion

The ECG shows progressive prolongation of the PR interval, with a P wave finally not conducted. There are actually two non-conducted P waves on this tracing. The first is the second P wave seen on the tracing (likely after progressive PR interval lengthening not pictured, but implied by the preceding long PR interval); the second is the seventh (which occurs after the progressive PR lengthening noted). This is consistent with Mobitz type I second-degree AV block.

Note the eye movements, lack of chin EMG signal and EEG waveforms consistent with REM sleep, which in some is a tonically cholinergic state. Note that no clear obstructive apnea is seen on this tracing.

Correct answer: C.

Discussion

The sleep-related rhythmic movement disorder or rhythmic movement disorder may also be called jactatio capitius nocturna or jactatio corporis nocturna.[1] In French, it is referred to as "rhythmie du sommeil." Rhythmic movement disorder refers not only to head banging but also to other repetitive stereotypic movements, including log-rolling, body rocking, leg banging, leg rolling, and head rolling. This type of behavior is most commonly seen in children, but the activity can persist into adulthood. It is most commonly seen during wakefulness prior to initial sleep onset, but may also be seen with nocturnal awakenings. The frequency is generally one movement per second, but can be seen with a frequency of one movement per 0.5 to 2 seconds

A. **Incorrect**. The respiratory pattern in this tracing is stable, and the patient is awake.
B. **Incorrect**. As above in A.
C. **Correct**. The most accurate answer is a sleep-related rhythmic movement disorder or rhythmic movement disorder. In the tracing, the signal that overwhelms the tracing originates from the LOC channel. The description of the epoch indicates that this occurred just after lights out and the patient is awake by the EEG tracing. By process of elimination, the correct answer is discernable. When the patient was viewed by video, he was in the left lateral position and was hitting his head against the pillow and headboard. The technologist appropriately documented the repetitive behavior.
D. **Incorrect**. There would be a chaotic movement pattern, not a rhythmic one as seen here.
E. **Incorrect**. The leg leads do show movement, but RLS is a clinical diagnosis, not one made based on a PSG. In addition, the most prominent finding is seen primarily in the LOC channel.

REFERENCE

1. American Academy of Sleep Medicine. *International Classification of Sleep Disorders, Diagnostic and Coding Manual*, 2nd edn. Westchester, IL: American Academy of Sleep Medicine, 2005.

Correct answer: E.

Discussion

The term "bigeminy" refers to a repetitive pattern of pairs of complexes. Ventricular bigeminy is not an uncommon finding in the sleep laboratory and consists of a repetitive sequence of one normal sinus impulse followed by one ventricular premature (wide) complex. Ventricular trigeminy is a repetitive sequence of two normal sinus impulses followed by one ventricular premature complex. Atrial bigeminy consists of a repetitive sequence of one normal sinus impulse followed by one atrial premature (narrow) complex.

A. **Incorrect**. The impulses are all narrow complex, but they are not regular in nature. Every other beat is premature, and there are no clear P waves preceding the QRS for the ectopic beats.

B. **Incorrect**. The impulses are not in the classic irregularly irregular pattern of atrial fibrillation. There is a "regular" pattern to the tracing. P waves are present before every other beat.

C. **Incorrect**. See all of the above. Further, classic flutter waves are not present.

D. **Incorrect**. There is a bigeminy pattern, but the premature beats are not wide complex.

E. **Correct**. Atrial bigeminy is rarely seen in the sleep laboratory. There is the repetitive sequence of one normal sinus impulse followed by one atrial premature (narrow) complex. Note that, just as in ventricular bigeminy, there is a constant interval between the normal beat and the subsequent premature beat and vice versa. Atrial bigeminy is usually a benign condition; however, patients (including the above patient) may complain of symptoms including palpitations.

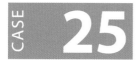

Correct answer: D.

Discussion

The respiratory finding is not considered pathologic. It is normal to see the respiratory volume decrease during bursts of phasic REM. The fall in volume will usually correspond to an increase in breathing rate in order to maintain the same minute ventilation.[1] These events are not scored as hypopneas unless there is an accompanying desaturation or arousal.[2]

A. **Incorrect**. The event does not meet criteria for an apnea (there is not a fall in the peak thermal sensor excursion by $\geq 90\%$ of baseline).[2]

B. **Incorrect**. There is clear effort in the thoracic and abdominal respiratory inductance plethysmography belts.

C. **Incorrect**. The event is not associated with a 3–4% desaturation or an arousal.[2]

E. **Incorrect**. The event does not meet criteria for an apnea, a hypopnea, or a RERA.[2]

REFERENCES

1. Guilleminault C. Sleep apnea syndromes: impact of sleep and sleep states. *Sleep* 1980;**3–4**:227–234.

2. Iber C, Ancoli-Israel S, Chesson A for the American Academy of Sleep Medicine. *The AASM Manual for the Scoring of Sleep and Associated Events: Rules, Terminology, and Technical Specifications*. Westchester, IL: American Academy of Sleep Medicine, 2007.

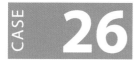

Question 1

Correct answer: E.

Discussion

A. **Accurate statement**. The bedtime is relatively consistent and is at midnight or later as indicated in the labeled bedtime in Fig. 2.

B. **Accurate statement**. Sleep-onset latency is variable as can be seen in the activity after bedtime; the patient clearly remains awake for several hours on 12/13/2010–12/15/2010, as noted in the red circles. There is much less activity after his bedtime on 12/16/2010, when the patient likely fell asleep relatively quickly.

C. **Accurate statement**. The time in bed is variable, which can be demonstrated by measuring the hours of rest for each day (from the bedtime to the out of bed time); the shortest appears to be on days 12/13/2010 and 12/17/2010. The longest appears to be on days 12/12/2010 and 12/16/2010.

D. **Accurate statement**. The out of bed time is variable, as indicated by the blue banner on Fig. 1. The earliest that the patient got out of bed was noon (12:00) on 12/13/2010, 12/15/10, and 12/17/10. The latest that the patient got out of bed was 4:00 p.m. (16:00) on 12/14/2010 and 12/16/2010.

E. **Inaccurate statement**. Once asleep, he does not have maintenance insomnia. On 12/17/2010, the patient clearly has several hours of wake time, as indicated by an increase in activity level. Please refer to the blue circle in Fig. 2

Question 2

Correct answer: B.

Discussion

A. **Incorrect**. The patient is experiencing a later bedtime and rise time than desired, not an earlier bedtime and rise time than desired.

B. **Correct**. The patient reports having difficulty initiating sleep at the desired time. He is able to achieve sleep at a later than desired time and sleep late into the morning (see the figures). This coincides with his report of not being sleepy at his goal bedtime but being able to "catch up" by sleeping in.

C. **Incorrect**. The history is not consistent with non-24 hour sleep–wake syndrome. In addition, the actigraphy tracing does not show a "free-running" pattern classically seen with this disorder.

D. **Incorrect**. The patient reports that his problem is a chronic one lasting 10 years and there is no mention of travel.

E. **Incorrect**. The actigraphy tracing is not consistent with a diagnosis of circadian rhythm disorder, irregular sleep–wake type, wherein an individual has lost the synchronizing effects of light, activity, and work/social activities. The individual in the current case clearly attempts to sleep at the same time every night.

CASE 27

Correct answer: D.

Discussion

A. **Correct statement**. The patient does sleep more than 8.5 hours per day on average, as indicated by the blue shaded areas. Each blue square is 1 hour; adding the night-time sleep opportunity to the napping gives the total sleep time for the day.

B. **Correct statement**. The patient took a nap at noon on day 2, day 3, and day 5. The patient took a nap at around 3:30 p.m. on day 6 and day 7.

C. **Correct statement**. The actigraphy monitor used for this study also has white light monitoring technology, as shown by the yellow line. White light is commonly represented in

this way, but there is also a legend that accompanies the tracing confirming this.

D. **Incorrect statement**. This is the one statement that is incorrect as the tracing here is a single plot tracing, with data for each day only represented one time. In addition, the time scale at the top and the bottom of the tracings confirm that this is a single plot actigraphy tracing (as they each show a 24 hour scale instead of a 48 hour scale).

E. **Correct statement**. The patient's bedtimes ranges from just before 20:00 (8:00 p.m.) on day 1 to just before 01:00 on day 2. The patient's wake time ranges from just before 06:00 (6:00 a.m.) on day 1, day 3, day 6, and day 7 to 08:30 (8:30 a.m.) on day 2.

CASE 28

Correct answer: D.

Discussion

A. **Incorrect**. While increased fraction of REM sleep, increased total REMs, and increased delta (N3) sleep have been shown with discontinuation of fluoxetine, REM latency would be expected to increase rather than decrease in this setting.[1]

B. **Incorrect**. Although decreased sleep latency and REM latency as well as increased N3 sleep can be seen in recovery sleep, increased REM sleep is not typically seen in recovery sleep after acute sleep deprivation unless there has been total sleep deprivation for greater than 60 hours.

C. **Incorrect**. Patients with narcolepsy have a short sleep latency and REM latency, but not increased stage N3 sleep or REM sleep fraction. Sleep fragmentation would also likely be seen in an overnight PSG of a patient with narcolepsy, which is not seen on this hypnogram.[2]

D. **Correct**. This hypnogram tracing, demonstrating relatively rapid sleep-stage cycling, short sleep and REM latencies, and a dominance of stage N3 sleep, is normal for a 4-month-old child referred for sleep-disordered breathing.[3]

E. **Incorrect**. Similar to the selective serotonin reuptake inhibitors (SSRIs), cocaine is a REM suppressant, and sleep during withdrawal will demonstrate an increased REM sleep percentage. However, there would likely be significant sleep fragmentation and there would not be a short REM latency, as seen here.

REFERENCES

1. Feige B, Voderholzer U, Reimann D, *et al*. Fluoxetine and sleep EEG: effects of a single dose, subchronic treatment, and discontinuation in healthy subjects. *Neuropsychopharmacology* 2002;**22**:246–258.

2. Aldrich MS. Diagnostic aspects of narcolepsy. *Neurology* 1998; **50**(Suppl 1):S2–S7.

3. Kahn A, Dan B, Groswasser J, *et al*. Normal sleep architecture in infants and children. *J Clin Neurophysiol* 1996;**13**:184–197.

Correct answer: C.

Discussion

A. **Incorrect**. According to the AASM pediatric scoring rules, an obstructive apnea must last for at least two breaths, be associated with > 90% fall in the thermal sensor amplitude, and have continued respiratory effort throughout the entire period.[1] In this example, although the thermal sensor amplitude is virtually absent, there is no associated respiratory effort.

B. **Incorrect**. A central apnea would be scored in a pediatric PSG if there was absent inspiratory effort for more than 20 seconds or lasting at least two breaths with an associated arousal, awakening, or 3% desaturation.[1] At least two of the events in this tracing do not have these associated findings.

C. **Correct**. In children, periodic breathing is defined as more than three episodes of central apnea lasting > 3 seconds and separated by no more than 20 seconds of normal breathing. It is more common in premature infants, decreasing with age, and is usually absent by age two years. Pediatric breathing has a more regular pattern during quiet sleep and is more irregular during active (REM) sleep (above). It was previously thought of as a predictor of sudden infant death syndrome, but that has been now shown not to be the case. It is considered to be a result of an immature brainstem.[2]

D. **Incorrect**. See C above.

E. **Incorrect**. Upper airway resistance syndrome is characterized by multiple arousals during sleep preceded by increased breathing effort without apnea or hypopnea. Esophageal pressure monitoring reveals multiple excessive breathing efforts terminated by arousals.[3]

REFERENCES

1. Iber C, Ancoli-Israel S, Chesson A for the American Academy of Sleep Medicine. *The AASM Manual for the Scoring of Sleep and Associated Events: Rules, Terminology, and Technical Specifications*. Westchester, IL: American Academy of Sleep Medicine, 2007.
2. Poets CF, Samuels MF, Southall DP. Epidemiology and pathophysiology of apnoea of prematurity. *Biol Neonate* 1994;**65**:211–219.
3. Guilleminault C, Stoohs R, Clerk A, *et al*. A cause of excessive daytime sleepiness: the upper airway resistance syndrome. *Chest* 1993;**104**:781–787.

Correct answer: B.

Discussion

A. **Incorrect**. See below.

B. **Correct**. Although short (3 seconds in duration), the respiratory event beginning at time marker 18 and ending at time marker 21 meets AASM criteria to score as an obstructive apnea in a pediatric patient. This event is associated with a > 90% fall in the thermal sensor for more than two breaths compared with the pre-event baseline amplitude.[1] This event is accompanied by severe O_2 desaturation, paradoxical thoracoabdominal respiratory effort, and loss of the capnography waveform, which are common in pediatric obstructive events. Note that there is a delay for both the capnometry and oximetry signals. Because of decreased functional residual volume and faster respiratory rate, children are more susceptible to gas exchange abnormalities from relatively brief respiratory events. Being a neonate with a congenitally small upper airway, this patient is especially susceptible to such changes.

C. **Incorrect**. Using the AASM pediatric scoring rules,[1] a hypopnea would be scored if there was a 50% drop in the amplitude of the nasal pressure signal lasting at least two breaths and accompanied by an arousal, awakening, or 3% desaturation. Because there is a > 90% fall in the thermal sensor (it is virtually flat), this event would be scored as an apnea rather than hypopnea.

D. **Incorrect**. A central apnea would be scored in a pediatric PSG for absent inspiratory effort for > 20 seconds or a shorter event of at least two breaths duration associated with an arousal, awakening, or 3% O_2 desaturation.[1] In this case, there is continued respiratory effort throughout the event.

E. **Incorrect**. The AASM recommends scoring a pediatric mixed apnea as an event that meets criteria for apnea and is associated with absent inspiratory effort in the initial part of the event, followed by resumption of the inspiratory effort before the event is over.[1] There is no absence of the initial respiratory effort in the event displayed in this case.

REFERENCE

1. Iber C, Ancoli-Israel S, Chesson A for the American Academy of Sleep Medicine. *The AASM Manual for the Scoring of Sleep and Associated Events: Rules, Terminology, and Technical Specifications*. Westchester, IL: American Academy of Sleep Medicine, 2007.

Correct answer: B.

Discussion

A. **Incorrect.** While insufficient EPAP could result in continued obstruction, this is not occurring in this tracing. There is not a 90% decrease in the airflow (in this case the PAP flow channel), which would be necessary by AASM criteria to score as apnea.[1] The lack of thoracoabdominal paradoxical breathing, which is often seen in pediatric obstructive apnea, also makes this interpretation less likely.

B. **Correct.** The PAP flow channel (from the PAP device pneumotachograph) shows the set bilevel ventilator back-up rate of 14 breaths/min. However, these mechanically ventilated breaths do not translate into movement of the patient's chest and abdomen, or $ETco_2$ waveforms. This poor triggering occurs when the inspiratory flow is insufficient to match inspiratory demand. It may be influenced by the amount of inspiratory time to reach the pressure target, the compliance and resistance of the respiratory circuit, and/or patient inspiratory effort.[2] Note that the capnography signal is distorted in this case by the high PAP pressures; consequently an end-tidal plateau is not obtained, making it inaccurate for assessing hypercapnia.

C. **Incorrect.** While there are few data establishing normal respiratory rates in sleeping children, a rate of 20–25 breaths/min would be normal for an awake 3 year old, and the respiratory rate would be lower during sleep.[3]

D. **Incorrect.** There would have to be a decrease in airflow of 50% or more for two breaths and an arousal, awakening, or desaturation of at least 3% to score a hypopnea by AASM criteria.[1]

REFERENCES

1. Iber C, Ancoli-Israel S, Chesson A for the American Academy of Sleep Medicine. *The AASM Manual for the Scoring of Sleep and Associated Events: Rules, Terminology, and Technical Specifications.* Westchester, IL: American Academy of Sleep Medicine, 2007.

2. Rabed C, Rodenstein D, Leger P, *et al.* Ventilator modes and settings during non-invasive ventilation: effects on respiratory events and implications for their identification. *Thorax* 2011;**66**:170–178.

3. Hooker EA, Danzl DF, Brueggmeyer M, Harper E. Respiratory rates in pediatric emergency patients. *J Emerg Med* 1992;**10**:407–410.

Question 1

Correct answer: D.

Discussion

A. **Incorrect.** Sleep-related oxygen desaturation in patients with COPD can occur in sleep *without* sleep apnea being present. Patients with COPD may or may not show signs of alveolar hypoventilation awake ($Pco_2 > 45$ mmHg) but will likely have exaggerated hypoventilation in sleep owing to the effects of NREM and REM sleep on the respiratory pump musculature. These patients may or may not have hypoxemia awake but often exhibit pronounced non-apneic desaturation in sleep related to lower lung O_2 stores and hypoventilation.

B. **Incorrect.** Oxygen supplementation may raise the saturation baseline awake and during some substages of sleep but may not be adequate when hypoventilation has reached a certain level of severity, especially in REM.

C. **Incorrect.** Bilevel PAP can augment tidal volumes and improve oxygenation as well as ventilation, but if emphysematous parenchymal disease is extensive, supplemental O_2 as well may be required to improve residual hypoxemia on bilevel PAP.

D. **Correct.**

Question 2

Correct answer: D.

Discussion

A. **Incorrect.** Such qualification is time consuming and requires several steps as outlined in the CMS national care determination policy.

B. **Incorrect.** An attended PSG must be performed and must determine that there is no OSA (AHI < 5/h), and thus that CPAP would not be indicated.

C. **Incorrect.** The patient must have oximetry in sleep showing that desaturation $< 88\%$ occurs for $\geqslant 5$ minutes on the usual Fio_2 or 2 L/min O_2, whichever is higher. The patient must be in a stable state on an adequate treatment regimen and demonstrate a persistent tendency to desaturate in sleep despite supplemental oxygen therapy.

D. **Correct.**

Further note: how is nocturnal oxyhemoglobin desaturation in sleep evaluated in a hypercarbic patient?

If a patient is hypercarbic, it is likely that oxyhemoglobin desaturation will accompany worsening hypoventilation in NREM and especially REM sleep, with atonia involving the respiratory pump muscles.

If this type of patient's history is positive for snoring, possible pauses in breathing in sleep and/or daytime sleepiness, then consideration should be given to evaluating for OSA apnea as an additional mechanism for sleep-related oxyhemoglobin desaturation.

The patient discussed in this case snored but did not have OSA. The snoring likely added some upper airway resistance to her work of breathing. The hypoventilation associated with her underlying COPD could then worsen in sleep to the point where simple O_2 supplementation could not help to maintain adequate saturation without further aggravating her hypercarbia and tendency towards respiratory acidosis.

A key point in qualifying patients with COPD who are on Medicare in the USA for non-invasive PAP based on the CMS criteria is that persistent desaturation has to be shown with $\geqslant 5$ minutes at $\leqslant 88\%$ on $\geqslant 2\,L/min\ O_2$. This requirement emphasizes the nature of the desaturations seen with hypoventilation, which cannot sometimes be treated with simple supplemental O_2 and may require assisted ventilation with or without supplemental O_2. A more commonly used standard for qualification for home O_2 therapy is that $\geqslant 5$ *cumulative* minutes of O_2 desaturation in sleep must be recorded. This different standard emphasizes the persistent and progressive nature of the desaturations seen with hypoventilation, which tend to be prolonged deep versus the rapid repetitive "sawtooth" desataration of OSA.

Although O_2 supplementation can be a reasonable treatment for many patients with COPD and nocturnal desaturation, later in the disease process more aggressive treatment with assisted ventilation is needed when O_2 alone is insufficient or possibly deleterious.

CASE 33

Correct answer: B.

Discussion

A. **Incorrect**. Although the differentiation between narcolepsy without cataplexy and idiopathic hypersomnia can be challenging, her history does offer some clues, including absence of frequent arousals, sense of non-refreshing naps, and long sleep times. Furthermore, no REM was seen during nap opportunities.

B. **Correct**. This patient's presenting history, sleep logs, overnight PSG study, and MSLT are consistent with idiopathic hypersomnia. She does not show the episodes of cataplexy, sleep paralysis, or hypnagogic hallucinations that would be consistent with narcolepsy with cataplexy. Her PSG and MSLT help to solidify the diagnosis. Her sleep architecture was normal, with generally decreasing blocks of N3 sleep with each cycle, and lengthening blocks of REM. On each MSLT nap opportunity, she fell asleep quickly (mean sleep onset 7.1 minutes), and entered NREM. She did not show REM sleep in any nap, nor did she demonstrate early-onset REM on the PSG. Idiopathic hypersomnia is characterized by excessive daytime sleepiness, with two forms distinguished: one with and the other without long sleep time > 10 hours. In idiopathic hypersomnia, sleep is typically characterized as non-refreshing, with significant sleep inertia or sleep "drunkenness." Similar to narcolepsy, the presentation is usually in young adulthood. Nocturnal sleep time is verified by PSG, which also excludes occult sleep-disordered breathing, PLMs, or other pathology. The MSLT is obtained to document daytime sleepiness and exclude SOREMs.

C. **Incorrect**. The patient's PSG and MSLT are consistent with insufficient sleep syndrome, but the history was deemed reliable and supported by sleep logs. Abundant N3 sleep could have suggested recovery sleep. Short latencies on the MSLT are a non-specific finding dependent on prior sleep behaviors. Actigraphy would have been a valuable additional diagnostic tool to monitor for insufficient sleep.

D. **Incorrect**. Delayed sleep phase disorder is an appropriate consideration because of the later wake-up times on weekends. Despite late sleep-onset times characteristic of this disorder, patients may successfully awaken for school and work commitments, although with great effort. These patients may then demonstrate excessive daytime sleepiness resulting from both circadian misalignment with the imposed wake schedule and chronic sleep deprivation from the shortened nocturnal sleep during the work week. In this case, the patient demonstrated no difficulty initiating sleep at early bedtimes and sleep logs showed no evidence of sleep deprivation. The MSLT in both delayed sleep phase disorder and sleep deprivation will typically show shorter sleep latencies in early naps compared with later ones. Analysis of circadian phase with measures of salivary dim-light melatonin onset may be appropriate when the diagnosis of phase delay is unclear.

E. **Incorrect**. There are no features of cataplexy, nor SOREMs on the MSLT.

Follow-up

After failing to respond to methylphenidate, the patient discontinued her oral contraceptive and was treated with modafinil. She reported an outstanding clinical response, with an easier time getting up in the morning, and much improved wakefulness during the day.

FURTHER READING
American Academy of Sleep Medicine. *International Classification of Sleep Disorders, Diagnostic and Coding Manual*, 2nd edn. Westchester, IL: American Academy of Sleep Medicine, 2005.

Morgenthaler TI, Kapur VK, Brown TM, *et al.* Practice parameters for the treatment of narcolepsy and other hypersomnias of central origin. *Sleep* 2007;**30**:1705–1711.

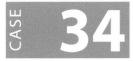

Correct answer: C.

Discussion

The patient's underlying primary pathology appears to be obstructive. His ethnic background, along with obesity, places him at particularly high risk of sleep-disordered breathing, given small caliber airway with narrowed anterior–posterior dimension.[1] The PSG is notable for respiratory events of variable length, relatively long in cycle nature, and the REM dominance of the disease, as demonstrated by severe desaturations that are more frequent events during REM (even on PAP during that time, as seen in the hypnogram).

Upon closer inspection of his hypnogram, however, there is clearly oximetry "banding" during NREM sleep. "Banding" is a term that can describe the pattern when desaturations are similar across a series of consecutive dips, and the compressed oximetry signal appears as a horizontal "band". Even though the respiratory events are obstructive, some of them have a self-similar, repetitive, short-cycle characteristic consistent with strong chemoreceptor modulation of control of breathing during NREM, presumably from chemoreceptor sensitization

in the setting of long-standing hypoxia. At the start of the desaturations, the desaturations are somewhat more irregular and then settle into the "band." Could this reflect induction of periodic breathing by the developing hypoxia? Notably, these events are fairly consistent in duration (metronomic), and snoring is only seen at time of arousal, as opposed to crescendo prior to arousal with classic obstructive disease. Both on the PSG and pathophysiologically, "mixed" events are common.

The patient was fortunate to have an apparent good response to CPAP overall (see Fig. 3 above) with few respiratory events and desaturations. There is a suggestion, as demonstrated in Fig. 3, that there is still some chemoreceptor influence, with somewhat prolonged unstable sleep–wake transitions and occasional post-arousal central apneas. The 10 minute epoch of wake to sleep transition shows a pattern continued for several minutes, with central apneas, post-arousal instability, and central apneas. Given that his primary pathology appears to be obstructive, however, "healing" of the chemoreceptor reflex should occur with time, as suggested by studies showing an improved NREM sleep CO_2 reserve following use of CPAP.[2]

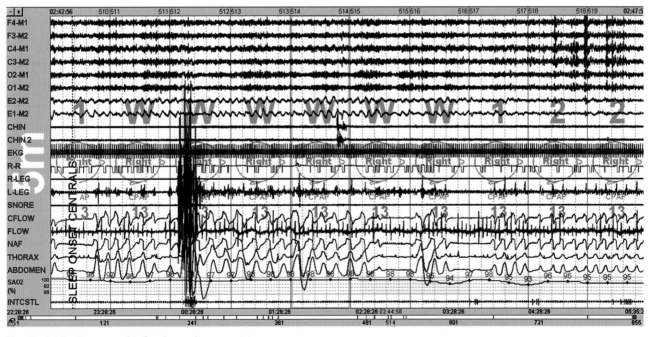

Fig. 3. A 10 minute epoch of wake to sleep transition.

REFERENCES

1. Lee RW, Vasudavan S, Hui DS, *et al*. Differences in craniofacial structures and obesity in Caucasian and Chinese patients with obstructive sleep apnea. *Sleep* 2010;**33**:1075–1080.

2. Imadojemu VA, Mawji Z, Kunselman A, *et al*. Sympathetic chemoreflex responses in obstructive sleep apnea and effects of continuous positive airway pressure therapy. *Chest* 2007;**131**:1406–1413.

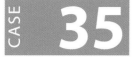

Correct answer: C.

Discussion

A. **Incorrect**. Periodic breathing was evident through the PAP trial.

B. **Incorrect**. Although there can be some transient bradypnea at initiation of PAP therapy, a prolonged event lasting greater than 2 minutes would not be consistent with this, nor would a central event during REM.

C. **Correct**. The patient demonstrated hypocapnia with dramatic induction of central apneas with application of CPAP. Periodic breathing was evident through the PAP trial. It is possible that his prior cerebrovascular accident may have played a role in enhanced chemoreceptor sensitivity or change in control of breathing, though more likely there was underlying hypocapnia. Looking back, it was evident on his diagnostic study that his events were NREM dominant, with virtually no respiratory disturbances during REM.

D. **Incorrect**. On the diagnostic study, initially the patient appeared to have purely obstructive disease, characterized by mostly obstructive hypopneic events with arousals and desaturations. Therefore, despite the fact that rates of sleep-disordered breathing are markedly higher in those who have had a cerebrovascular accident, it is unlikely that this alone contributed to centrally mediated events in this man, as one would expect those to be seen on the diagnostic study; the appearance is also not consistent with Cheyne–Stokes breathing.

Follow-up

The patient returned for a "complex" titration study, completed with $ETco_2$ monitoring, which confirmed hypocapnia, in the 36 mmHg range, during NREM. Application of enhanced expiratory rebreathing space, a non-vented mask, and supplemental O_2 much improved the response to CPAP, as seen in Fig. 4 (above) during stage N2 sleep. Acetazolamide could also be considered should the patient have an incomplete response.

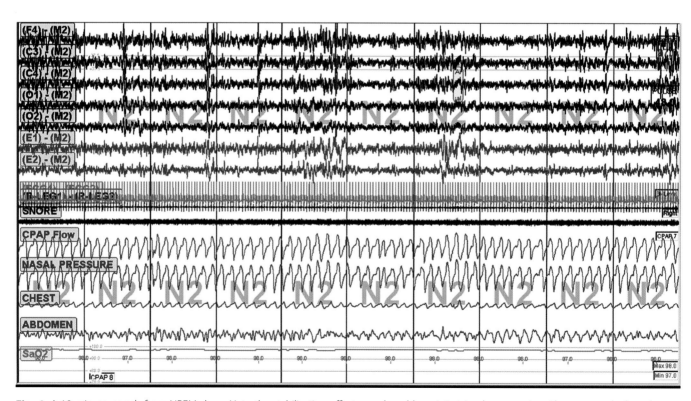

Fig. 4. A 10 minute epoch from NREM sleep. Note the stabilization effects produced by minimizing hypocapnia with a non-vented mask, and hypoxia with supplemental O_2.

FURTHER READING
Gilmartin G, McGeehan B, Vigneault K, *et al.* Treatment of positive airway pressure treatment-associated respiratory instability with enhanced expiratory rebreathing space (EERS). *J Clin Sleep Med* 2010;**6**:529–538.

Parra O, Arboix A, Bechich S, *et al.* Time course of sleep-related breathing disorders in first-ever stroke or transient ischemic attack. *Am J Respir Crit Care Med* 2000;**161**:375–380.

CASE 36

Correct answer: B.

Discussion

This patient demonstrates abnormal bradypnea during the course of his sleep study with a somewhat ataxic appearance and a significant number of centrally mediated events. He was not using opiates. While there was mild obstructive sleep-disordered breathing, mainly comprising flow limitation during stable sleep (Fig. 1), the dysrhythmic breathing was not typical of OSA alone.

A. **Incorrect.** See B below.

B. **Correct.** Before embarking on possible remedial steps, it would be prudent to use an MRI evaluation to ensure that an Arnold–Chiari malformation does not exist. This patient's MRI showed such a malformation. An Arnold–Chiari malformation radiologically shows an elongation of the cerebellar tonsils below the foramen magnum; there are several different types characterized. Though exact numbers are unknown, it is felt to be symptomatic in 1 in 1000 patients. The association between sleep-disordered breathing, particularly central apnea syndromes, has been long described in the literature, particularly in younger patients. The mechanism by which the malformation contributes to pathologic sleep breathing may be through compression of brainstem structures involved in control of breathing, or through associated developmental abnormalities.

C. **Incorrect.** A hypnotic medication may minimize arousals from sleep but would not address the irregular breathing pattern seen above.

D. **Incorrect.** See B above.

Follow-up

The patient was referred for neurosurgical consultation based on the identification of the Arnold–Chiari malformation. The key point here is that ataxic respiration or central apneas in a young individual should raise the suspicion of a craniovertebral junction abnormality. The features of the tracing may not be adequately captured by the traditional AHI. Once a cause has been identified, lateral sleep, weight loss, and a possible CPAP trial may all be appropriate.

FURTHER READING
Balk RA, Hiller FC, Lucas EA, *et al.* Sleep apnea and the Arnold–Chiari malformation. *Am Rev Respir Dis* 1985;**132**:929–930.
Dauvilliers Y, Stal V, Abril B, *et al.* Chiari malformation and sleep-related breathing disorders. *J Neurol Neurosurg Psychiatry* 2007;**78**:1344–1348.
Zolty P, Sanders MH, Pollack IF. Chiari malformation and sleep-disordered breathing: a review of diagnostic and management issues. *Sleep* 2000;**23**:637–643.

CASE 37

Correct answer: C.

Discussion

A. **Incorrect.** The lateral and posterior hypothalamus is an area producing hypocretins, among other roles, and is not involved in the generation of sleep spindles.

B. **Incorrect.** The locus coeruleus is primarily responsible for the production of the neurotransmitter norepinephrine and stress responses. It is not involved in the generation of sleep spindles.

C. **Correct.** The finding marked by the arrow is a sleep spindle, which is characterized by a train of distinct waves with a frequency of 11–16 Hz (most commonly 12–14 Hz) and a duration of ≥ 0.5 seconds. Spindles are generated by the thalamic reticular nuclei and are maximally seen in the central leads. Stage N2 sleep is, in part, defined by the presence of sleep spindles and/or K-complexes without arousals. While characteristic of stage N2 sleep, sleep spindles may also occur in stages N3 and REM sleep. They first appear during the initial 1 to 2 months of life, decrease in density with advancing age in both men and women, and may be affected by benzodiazepines, which may increase spindle density, frequency, and duration.

D. **Incorrect.** The pineal gland is mainly responsible for the production of melatonin.

E. **Incorrect.** The tubomammillary nucleus is a histamine-producing area associated with the control of arousal, sleep and circadian rhythm; however, it is not involved in the generation of sleep spindles.

161

FURTHER READING
Crowley K, Trinder J, Kim Y, Carrington M, Colrain IM. The effects of normal aging on sleep spindle and K-complex production. *Clin Neurophysiol* 2002;**113**:1615–1622.

McCormick L, Nielsen T, Nicolas A, *et al.* Topographical distribution of spindles and K-complexes in normal subjects. *Sleep* 1997;**20**:939–941.
Silber MH, Ancoli-Israel S, Bonnet MH, *et al.* The visual scoring of sleep in adults. *J Clin Sleep Med* 2007;**3**:121–132.

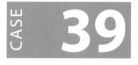

Correct answer: B.

Discussion

An MSLT nap session may be terminated by any of three clearly defined events. If no sleep occurs during a given trial, the trial is terminated after 20 minutes with the sleep latency value being calculated as 20 minutes. In trials where sleep occurs prior to reaching the 20 minute trial limit, the sleep latency is calculated as the time from lights out to any stage of sleep, including stage N1 sleep. If NREM sleep occurs during a given nap, the trial is permitted to continue for up to 15 minutes of clock time to observe for the onset of REM sleep. If REM sleep is observed during this period, the REM latency is calculated as the time from the first epoch of sleep to the first epoch of REM sleep, regardless of intervening sleep stages or wakefulness. The trial is terminated once the first epoch of REM sleep occurs. If REM sleep does not occur within 15 minutes after the initial onset NREM sleep, the trial is also terminated.

A. **Incorrect**. Epoch A represents NREM stage N2 sleep as evidenced by the presence of sleep spindles and K-complexes.

B. **Correct**. Given the rules for MSLT trial termination, the trial in the given case should be terminated after epoch B, which represents stage REM sleep. The REM sleep in epoch B is characterized by low-voltage mixed frequency EEG activity with episodic REMs and reduced chin EMG activity.

C. **Incorrect**. Epoch C represents NREM stage N1 sleep, as evidenced by the presence of low-amplitude mixed frequency activity occupying > 50% of the epoch. Note that the activity seen in the EOG channels is slow rolling eye movement activity rather than REM activity as seen in epoch B.

D. **Incorrect**. Epoch D represents NREM stage N3 sleep, as more than 20% of the given epoch consists of slow wave activity.

FURTHER READING
Iber C, Ancoli-Israel S, Chesson A for the American Academy of Sleep Medicine. *The AASM Manual for the Scoring of Sleep and Associated Events: Rules, Terminology, and Technical Specifications.* Westchester, IL: American Academy of Sleep Medicine, 2007.
Littner M, Kushida C, Wise M, *et al.* Practice parameters for clinical use of the Multiple Sleep Latency Test and the Maintenance of Wakefulness Test. *Sleep* 2005;**28**:113–144.

Correct answer: D.

Discussion

The MSLT is a validated test for the assessment of objective sleepiness and is indicated in clinical practice as part of the evaluation of patients with suspected narcolepsy or idiopathic hypersomnia. Since there are several etiologies that may cause daytime sleepiness, strict adherence to the MSLT protocol is critical. According to the 2005 AASM practice parameters for the clinical use of the MSLT and the maintenance of wakefulness test (MWT),[1] the MSLT should be performed on the day following an overnight PSG, with the preceding overnight PSG having a minimum total sleep time of at least 6 hours.

A. **Incorrect**. This would not be advisable given the available data, especially in the absence of cataplexy.

B. **Incorrect**. This would not be advisable given the available data, especially in the absence of cataplexy.

C. **Incorrect**. Given the absence of PSG data to support a diagnosis of OSA, there is no information to support the recommendation for a CPAP titration study.

D. **Correct**. Based on the history and data presented in this case, therefore, and despite the findings of a very low mean sleep-onset latency and the presence of three REM periods on the MSLT, there are in fact insufficient data to make a reliable clinical decision. Specifically, given the absence of PSG data from the night prior to the MSLT, the MSLT results by themselves cannot be reliably interpreted. Note that the MSLT by itself is diagnostic of nothing and cannot be interpreted in isolation. The results of the MSLT must be interpreted in the context of the entire clinical presentation and only supports a diagnosis of narcolepsy or idiopathic hypersomnia in the proper clinical setting. Even the presence of multiple SOREM periods, as seen here, is not specific for narcolepsy, as this finding may be seen in 3–17% of the general population.[2]

REFERENCES
1. Littner M, Kushida C, Wise M, *et al*. Practice parameters for clinical use of the Multiple Sleep Latency Test and the Maintenance of Wakefulness Test. *Sleep* 2005;**28**:113–144.

2. Singh M, Drake CL, Roth T. The prevalence of multiple sleep-onset REM periods in a population based sample. *Sleep* 2006;**29**:890–895.

CASE 40

Correct answer: C.

Discussion

The example demonstrates absence of the nasal pressure flow signal because of a malfunction of the nasal pressure sensor. Nasal pressure monitoring is currently the recommended method for measuring hypopneas and flow limitation. Several studies have shown that nasal pressure monitoring has a strong correlation with the gold standard, pneumotachography, and is superior to thermistor monitoring for the measurement and detection of hypopneas.

While nasal pressure monitoring is the preferred method for monitoring hypopneas, it is not sensitive enough for measuring the absence of airflow (e.g. the patient may be mouth breathing) and is, therefore, not the recommended method for the measurement of apneas. Thermal sensors offer a more reliable method for measuring apneas, but are inadequate for measuring lesser reductions in airflow such as hypopneas and flow limitation events. Given the strengths and limitations of these two types of sensor, the current AASM Manual recommends nasal pressure monitoring for the assessment of hypopneas and nasal/oro-thermistor measurement for the assessment of apneas.

A. **Incorrect**. This choice is incorrect as the thermistor signal is functioning appropriately. Thermal sensor measurement is a reliable method for measuring the absence of airflow and is currently the recommended method for measuring apneas.

B. **Incorrect**. This answer is incorrect as there are no problems with the EEG signals and, therefore, the arousal index should not be affected.

C. **Correct**. Given the absence of the nasal pressure signal, this study would be expected to underestimate the number of hypopneas and, therefore, potentially underestimate both the AHI and respiratory disturbance index.

D. **Incorrect**. The absence of the nasal pressure signal should result in a reduction in the numbers of measured hypopneas and, therefore, an underestimation of the AHI.

FURTHER READING
Iber C, Ancoli-Israel S, Chesson A for the American Academy of Sleep Medicine. *The AASM Manual for the Scoring of Sleep and Associated Events: Rules, Terminology, and Technical Specifications*. Westchester, IL: American Academy of Sleep Medicine, 2007.

Heitman S, Atkar R, Hajduk E, *et al*. Validation of nasal pressure for the identification of apneas/hypopneas during sleep. *Am J Respir Crit Care Med* 2002;**166**:386–391.

Redline S, Budhiraja R, Kapur V, *et al*. Reliability and validity of respiratory event measurement and scoring. *J Clin Sleep Med* 2007;**3**:169–200.

CASE 41

Correct answer: C.

Discussion

According to the 2005 AASM practice parameters for the clinical use of the MSLT and MWT,[1] the termination of an MWT trial occurs after 40 minutes of no sleep or after unequivocal sleep, which is defined as three consecutive epochs of stage N1 sleep or one epoch of any other stage of sleep. The sleep latency for a given MWT trial is calculated from lights out to the onset of unequivocal sleep or after 40 minutes of no sleep.

The definition for sleep latency and trial termination differs between the MWT and MSLT. The sleep latency for the MSLT is calculated as the time from lights out to any stage of sleep, including stage 1. Also, once sleep onset has been achieved on the MSLT, the test is continued for 15 minutes of clock time to observe for SOREM periods. By comparison, once unequivocal sleep has been achieved on the MWT, the trial is terminated. The occurrence of REM sleep on the MWT is not important to the utility of the test.

A. **Incorrect**. Epoch A represents stage wake.

B. **Incorrect**. Epoch B represents stage N1 sleep. The sleep latency and termination definition for the MWT require the presence of unequivocal sleep. One epoch of stage N1 sleep does not meet the sleep latency definition.

C. **Correct**. Epoch C represents stage N2 sleep. Given the recommended trial termination definition for the MWT, the trial here should be terminated after epoch C, as stage N2 sleep is the first epoch of sleep that meets the definition of unequivocal sleep.

D. **Incorrect**. Epoch D represents stage N3 sleep. Given that these examples represent consecutive epochs, choice D is incorrect as the trial would have been terminated after unequivocal sleep was observed in epoch C with stage N2 sleep.

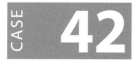

REFERENCE
1. Littner M, Kushida C, Wise M, *et al*. Practice parameters for clinical use of the Multiple Sleep Latency Test and the Maintenance of Wakefulness Test. *Sleep* 2005;**28**:113–144.

Correct answer: A.

Discussion

This PSG tracing demonstrates slow-wave activity throughout the majority of the epoch, meeting the definition of stage N3 sleep. Stage N3 sleep is scored when 20% or more of an epoch consists of slow-wave activity, irrespective of the individual's age. Slow-wave activity is defined by waves in the frequency range 0.5–2 Hz and a peak-to-peak amplitude of > 75 µV, measured over the frontal regions. An earlier set of scoring criteria subdivided slow-wave sleep into stages 3 and 4 sleep based on the percentage of a given epoch with slow-wave activity. A review of the literature and consensus opinion found no validity or biological significance to this subdivision and the current AASM Manual only recognizes stage N3 sleep as defined above.

A. **Correct**. Stage N3 sleep typically occurs in the first third of the night and is tightly linked to the release of growth hormone.
B. **Incorrect**. Stage N3 sleep typically occurs in the first third of the night, not the second half.

C. **Incorrect**. Unlike REM sleep, which is primarily mediated by circadian processes, increases in slow-wave sleep activity are primarily driven by the homeostatic sleep mechanism, with increases in stage N3 sleep being observed after acute sleep deprivation and reductions observed after recovery sleep.
D. **Incorrect**. Slow-wave sleep, as a percentage of the total sleep time, is greatest in young children and becomes less common with advancing age.
E. **Incorrect**. Tricyclic antidepressants, like most antidepressant medications, are suppressants of stage REM sleep, not stage N3 sleep.

FURTHER READING
Carskadon M, Dement W. Normal human sleep: an overview. In *Principles and Practice of Sleep Medicine*, 5th edn, Kryger M, Roth T, Dement W (eds.). St Louis, MO: Elsevier Saunders, 2011, pp. 16–26.
Silber MH, Ancoli-Israel S, Bonnet MH, *et al*. The visual scoring of sleep in adults. *J Clin Sleep Med* 2007;**3**:121–132.
Van Cauter E, Plat L, Copinschi G. Interrelations between sleep and the somatotropic axis. *Sleep* 1998;**21**:553–566.

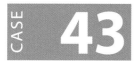

Correct answer: A.

The ECG finding is most consistent with atrial fibrillation. Atrial fibrillation, as demonstrated in this example, is characterized by an irregularly irregular pattern of RR intervals and the absence of P waves. Although the atrial activity may at first be thought to represent flutter rather than fibrillation, the irregularity of the waves and QRS rhythm is more characteristic of atrial fibrillation than atrial flutter.

A. **Correct**. Several studies have demonstrated that atrial fibrillation as well other arrhythmias, including complex ventricular ectopy and non-sustained supraventricular tachycardia, have an increased prevalence in patients with OSA compared with age-matched controls. The risk of atrial fibrillation in patients with OSA is particularly high in those individuals with more severe nocturnal hypoxemia.
B. **Incorrect**. The prevalence and incidence of atrial fibrillation increase with age and with underlying heart disease. In patients under the age of 60 years, there appears to be a circadian variation in the incidence of paroxysmal atrial

fibrillation with an increased incidence between the hours of 12 midnight and 5 a.m. This circadian distribution is not seen in those over the age of 60.
C. **Incorrect**. While non-randomized observational studies suggest that CPAP therapy may reduce the recurrence of atrial fibrillation in those who have undergone electrical cardioversion, there are currently no large-scale randomized controlled data to support CPAP as a treatment that consistently resolves or improves atrial fibrillation.
D. **Incorrect**. Most studies have demonstrated that concomitant atrial fibrillation in the presence of congestive heart failure has been associated with *increased* morbidity and mortality.

FURTHER READING
Mehra R, Benjamin E, Gottlieb D, *et al*. Association of nocturnal arrythmias with sleep-disordered breathing: The sleep heart health study. *Am J Respir Crit Care Med* 2006;**173**:910–916.
Olsson LG, Swedberg K, Ducharme A, *et al*. Atrial fibrillation and risk of clinical events in chronic heart failure with and without left ventricular

systolic dysfunction: Results of the Candesartan in Heart failure-Assessment of Reduction in Mortality and Morbidity (CHARM) program. *J Am Coll Cardiol* 2006;**47**:1997–2004.

Yamashita T, Murakawa Y, Hayami N, *et al.* Relation between aging and circadian variation of paroxysmal atrial fibrillation. *Am J Cardiol* 1998;**82**:1364–1367.

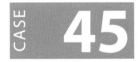

Correct answer: B.

Discussion

Normal gastrointestinal physiology during sleep is characterized by decreases in swallowing rate, salivary production, and esophageal and intestinal motility. There is also a circadian rhythm in basal gastric acid secretion, with the peak secretion occurring between 10 p.m. and 2 a.m. In those individuals who suffer from gastroesophageal reflux during sleep, episodes most commonly occur during stage N2 sleep, mainly after brief awakenings or arousals.

A. **Incorrect**. Epoch A represents stage N1 sleep, which is characterized by low-amplitude mixed frequency activity occupying more than 50% of the epoch.
B. **Correct**. Epoch B represents stage N2 sleep, given the presence of both sleep spindles and K-complexes without associated arousals occurring in the first half of the epoch.

C. **Incorrect**. Epoch C represents stage N3 sleep, which demonstrates slow-wave activity occupying more than 20% of the given epoch. In this example, the slow-wave activity occupies almost the entirety of epoch C.
D. **Incorrect**. This represents stage REM sleep. This example shows rapid conjugate, irregular eye movements associated with low-amplitude mixed frequency activity and low EMG chin tone. Eye movement artifacts are demonstrated in the frontal leads, as well as the central leads but to a lesser extent.

FURTHER READING

Orr WC, Heading R, Johnson LF, *et al.* Sleep and its relationship with gastroesophageal reflux. *Aliment Pharmacol Ther* 2004;**9**(Suppl):39–46.

Gerson LB, Fass R. A systematic review of the definitions, prevalence, and response to treatment of nocturnal gastroesophageal reflux disease. *Clin Gastroenterol Hepatol* 2009;**7**:372–378.

Penzel T, Becker HR, Brandenburg U, *et al.* Arousals in patients with gastroesophageal reflux and sleep apnea. *Eur Respir J* 1999;**14**:1266–1277.

Correct answer: D.

Discussion

The finding identified in this epoch is most consistent with the alpha EEG sleep pattern. The alpha EEG pattern, which has also been termed alpha intrusion sleep and alpha–delta sleep patterns, is characterized by abnormal alpha wave activity during NREM stages 2 and 3 sleep. This alpha activity during NREM sleep tends to be somewhat slower than alpha activity observed during wakefulness (7–12 Hz) and may be best observed over the frontal leads (although it is represented in all the derivations in the current tracing). While a formal classification system for this EEG pattern does not currently exist, studies of EEG frequency analysis have attempted to categorize the alpha EEG sleep pattern into three distinct types: (1) tonic alpha EEG sleep occurring throughout NREM stages 2 and 3 with > 40% of the EEG having the alpha frequency; (2) phasic alpha EEG sleep, in which the alpha EEG pattern occurs predominantly during NREM stage 3 sleep (alpha–delta sleep pattern); and (3) periodic K-complex–alpha and periodic polyphasic EEG burst activity.

A. **Incorrect**. Fibromyalgia is diagnosed by clinical criteria as outlined by the American College of Rheumatology. Sleep complaints, or specific findings on an overnight PSG, including the alpha EEG sleep pattern, are not required for a diagnosis.
B. **Incorrect**. While the alpha EEG sleep pattern has been described in association with fibromyalgia, it is neither a sensitive nor a specific finding for the diagnosis of this or any condition. It has been observed in association with several chronic diseases, such as rheumatoid arthritis and other chronic pain syndromes, and has also been observed in normal individuals.
C. **Incorrect**. While some studies have shown a relationship between the alpha EEG pattern and increased daytime fatigue, the presence of the alpha EEG pattern in patients with fibromyalgia has not been consistently demonstrated to correlate with symptom severity.
D. **Correct**. Recent studies evaluating the use of sodium oxybate in patients with fibromyalgia have demonstrated a reduction in the alpha EEG pattern in addition to increased slow-wave sleep activity and improved daytime symptoms. The mechanisms by which sodium oxybate may be responsible for these outcomes are not clear.

FURTHER READING

Maclean AW, Lue F, Moldofsky H. The reliability of visual scoring of alpha EEG activity during sleep. *Sleep* 1995;**18**:565–569.

Moldofsky H, Inhaber NH, Guinta DR, Alvarez-Horine SB. Effects of sodium oxybate on sleep physiology and sleep–wake-related symptoms in patients with fibromyalgia syndrome: A double-blind, randomized, placebo-controlled study. *J Rheumatol* 2010;**37**:2156–2166.

Scharf M, Baumann M, Berkowitz DV. The effects of sodium oxybate on clinical symptoms and sleep patterns in patients with fibromyalgia. *J Rheumatol* 2003;**30**:1070–1074.

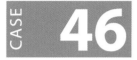

Correct answer: D.

Discussion

Short irregular bursts of transient muscle activity may be observed in normal REM sleep. These normal transient muscle bursts are typically of short duration (< 0.25 seconds); may been seen in the chin and limb EMG, EOG and/or EEG leads; and are typically associated with REM (phasic REM sleep). In this example, however, REM sleep is associated with excessive muscle activity in both the lower extremity limb EMG and the chin EMG leads during both tonic and phasic REM sleep. These findings are most consistent with REM sleep without atonia.

Occurrence of REM sleep without atonia has been described in association with RBD, narcolepsy, neurodegenerative disorders such as Parkinson's disease and Lewy body dementia, and in association with certain medications including most classes of antidepressants and L-DOPA.

The PSG finding of REM sleep without atonia is not sufficient alone to make a diagnosis of RBD. This is the only parasomnia that requires a PSG to confirm its diagnosis. The ICSD-2 criteria for the diagnosis of RBD include: (1) the presence of REM sleep without atonia; (2) a history of sleep-related injurious or potentially injurious behaviors or abnormal REM sleep behaviors documented during PSG monitoring; and (3) the absence of EEG epileptiform activity during REM sleep.

A. **Incorrect**. Clonazepam has been used successfully in the treatment of RBD but is not indicated in this case as noted above.

B. **Incorrect**. Melatonin has been used successfully in the treatment of RBD but is not indicated in this case as noted above.

C. **Incorrect**. Venlafaxine is not indicated for RBD or REM sleep without atonia and may, in fact, increase the severity of these events.

D. **Correct**. The patient in this example demonstrates REM sleep without atonia but does not meet the other ICSD-2 diagnostic criteria for the diagnosis of RBD, given the absence of abnormal or injurious behavior by history and the absence of abnormal behaviors in REM sleep during PSG. In the absence of RBD, REM sleep without atonia alone does not require treatment.

FURTHER READING

Aurora R, Zak R, Maganti R, *et al*. Best practice for the treatment of REM sleep behavior disorder (RBD). *J Clin Sleep Med* 2010;**6**:85–95.

Walters A, Lavigne G, Hening W, *et al*. The scoring of movements in sleep. *J Clin Sleep Med* 2007;**3**:155–167.

Winkelman JW, James L. Serotonergic antidepressants are associated with REM sleep without atonia. *Sleep* 2004;**27**:317–321.

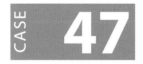

Correct answer: B.

Discussion

A. **Incorrect**. Although opening the tracheostomy would treat the OSA, many such patients and especially school-aged children hope for decannulation after diaphragmatic pacing is initiated.

B. **Correct**. Upper airway obstruction can occur during sleep with paced breaths when the diaphragm contracts without a centrally coordinated effort to maintain airway patency. The activation of the upper airway and laryngeal muscles is necessary to counteract the negative pharyngeal pressure generated during inspiration.[1] Lowering the amplitude would help in alleviating the obstructive events by improving the pressure differential across the luminal wall.[2] Another way to avoid airway occlusion is to increase the inspiratory time on the pacer. The clinician must also ensure that the hypoventilation is adequately treated and if necessary minute ventilation can be increased by increasing the rate of the pacing rather than the amplitude of the stimuli.

C. **Incorrect**. While such therapy might treat the obstructive apneas, as well as provide ventilatory support, the main goal of diaphragmatic pacing is to move away from both invasive and non-invasive mechanical ventilation.

D. **Incorrect.** Waking the patient repeatedly might treat the OSA, but would also produce diminished sleep quality and a very tired family. Unlike other conditions in which an obstructive apnea with hypercapnia would lead to an arousal, patients with central congenital hypoventilation syndrome rarely have arousals even with profound hypercapnia.

E. **Incorrect.** Although changing the patient's position from supine to lateral decubitus may improve the obstructive events somewhat, this patient would most likely continue to have sleep-disordered breathing.[3]

REFERENCES
1. Ilbawi MN, Idriss FS, Hunt CE, *et al.* Diaphragmatic pacing in infants: techniques and results. *Ann Thorac Surg* 1985;**40**:323–329.
2. Chen ML, Tablizo MA, Kun S, Keens TG. Diaphragm pacers as a treatment for congenital central hypoventilation syndrome. *Expert Rev Med Devices* 2005;**2**:577–585.
3. Dayyat E, Maarafeya MMA, Capdevila OS, *et al.* Nocturnal body position in sleeping children with and without obstructive sleep apnea. *Pediatr Pulmonol* 2007;**42**:374–379.

CASE 48

Correct answer: D.

Discussion

A. **Incorrect.** Close inspection of the pressure channel shows that the patient is frequently not triggering the IPAP–EPAP cycle. Although widening the pressure differential by increasing the pressure support improves tidal volume and may improve hypoventilation somewhat, if the patient is not able to trigger the IPAP–EPAP cycle, gains from higher IPAP would be limited.

B. **Incorrect.** While improving the mask leak is helpful in general, particularly in situations when the patient fails to trigger the ventilator, and this answer could seem appropriate because of the air leak, the leak here is not unusual for these relatively high PAP settings.

C. **Incorrect.** Bilevel PAP generates higher tidal volumes by virtue of pressure support,[1] and uncontrolled administration of CPAP may be harmful in some patients with kyphoscoliosis. This is because extreme stiffness of the chest wall can lead to increased functional residual capacity.[2]

D. **Correct.** Children with neuromuscular diseases and restrictive lung diseases are not always able to trigger the IPAP–EPAP cycle on the bilevel PAP and the addition of a back-up rate is helpful. The AASM recommends pressure support between 4 and 20 cmH$_2$O and the use of spontaneous timed or timed mode, starting at a rate equal to or slightly less than the patient's spontaneous sleeping respiratory rate.[3]

E. **Incorrect.** The ET$_{CO_2}$ values continue to be excessive, and the patient is not able to trigger the IPAP–EPAP cycle. Chronic hypoventilation is associated with life-threatening conditions such as pulmonary hypertension and cor pulmonale, and is also associated with chronic hypoxemia and polycythemia.[2] Sufficient evidence exists to support the use of non-invasive positive pressure ventilation through a mask during sleep.[3]

REFERENCES
1. Becker HF, Piper AJ, Flynn WE, *et al.* Breathing during sleep in patients with nocturnal desaturation. *Am J Respir Crit Care Med* 1999;**159**:112–118.
2. Kryger MH. Restrictive lung disorders. In *Principles and Practice of Sleep Medicine*, 4th edn, Kryger M, Roth T, Dement W (eds.). Philadelphia, PA: Saunders, 2005, pp.1136–1144.
3. Berry RB, Chediak A, Brown LK, *et al.* Best clinical practices for the sleep center adjustment of non-invasive positive pressure ventilation (NPPV) in stable chronic alveolar hypoventilation syndromes. *J Clin Sleep Med* 2010;**6**:491–509.

CASE 49

Correct answer: B

A. **Incorrect.** These epochs show N3 sleep, which has a frequency of 0.5–2 Hz with amplitude of 75 μV shown here and is enhanced from the first to the second tracing. Fast frequencies such as beta rhythm have a frequency over 13 Hz. Benzodiazepines have been shown to increase beta frequency and sleep spindles.[1]

B. **Correct.** In this example, there is increased density and amplitude of slow waves in Fig. 1B compared with the earlier slow-wave sleep (Fig. 1B); this is not normal sleep architecture as slow-wave sleep predominantly occurs early in the night. Sodium oxybate (Xyrem) is approved for the treatment of cataplexy and excessive daytime sleepiness from narcolepsy. Sodium oxybate has a short half-life (30–60 minutes) and is taken at bedtime, with the second dose 2.5–4 hours later. Its mechanism of action to improve daytime sleepiness is not known. Studies show an increase in the mean sleep latency on the MWT from 5.5 minutes to 10.6 minutes (9 g dose) and a decrease in the Epworth Sleepiness Scale score from 19 to 12.[2,3] Sodium oxybate increases slow-wave sleep and delta power, and decreases nocturnal arousals; this effect is dose dependent and is seen at doses of 7.5–9 g.

C. **Incorrect**. REM sleep has a low-amplitude mixed frequency EEG. Although REM sleep can rebound after sleep deprivation, no such rebound is depicted here.

D. **Incorrect**. Please see answer A.

E. **Incorrect**. The EEG shows enhanced N3 sleep, but zolpidem suppresses N3 sleep. The factors that can enhance slow-wave sleep include sleep deprivation, illness, exercise, and medications including sodium oxybate, gabapentin, tiagabine, and gaboxadol.

REFERENCES

1. Aeschbach D, Dijk DJ, Trachsel L, Brunner DP, Borbely AA. Dynamics of slow-wave activity and spindle frequency activity in the human sleep EEG: effect of midazolam and zopiclone. *Neuropsychopharmacology* 1994;**11**:237–244.

2. Mamelak M, Black J, Montplaisir J, Ristanovic R. A pilot study on the effects of sodium oxybate on sleep architecture and daytime alertness in narcolepsy. *Sleep* 2004;**27**:1327–1334.

3. Xyrem International Study G. A double-blind, placebo-controlled study demonstrates sodium oxybate is effective for the treatment of excessive daytime sleepiness in narcolepsy. *J Clin Sleep Med* 2005;**1**:391–397.

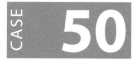

CASE 50

Correct answer: A.

Discussion

A. **Correct**. Most opioids are selective for the μ receptor. Opioids cause a blunted central chemosensitivity to hypercapnia through a direct action of the μ receptor on the brainstem respiratory centers.[1,2]

B. **Incorrect**. Central sleep apnea is found in a far lower percentage of such patients; for example, 30% of subjects on chronic methadone were shown to have such central sleep apnea.[3]

C. **Incorrect**. In the acute and chronic phase, opioids reduce REM and slow-wave (N3) sleep.

D. **Incorrect**. The tracing shows repetitive central apneas: absence of thermal sensor excursion with absent inspiratory effort. Cheyne–Stokes breathing consists of cyclical crescendo–decrescendo breathing, with the central apnea characteristically occurring at the nadir of the waning breathing effort. Such breathing is not clearly displayed here, where the apneas appear more abruptly than typical for Cheyne–Stokes breathing. Further, this setting is not consistent with a diagnosis of Cheyne–Stokes breathing pattern under current ICSD-2 criteria, which requires a serious underlying medical illness and the absence of medications that could otherwise better explain such breathing. However, it should be noted that crescendo–decrescendo breathing can sometimes be seen with opioid-induced central sleep apnea.[4]

E. **Incorrect**. In general, opioids cause greater reductions in respiratory rate rather than tidal volume.[1,2]

Follow-up

A repeat study carried out 1 year later, when the woman was off all medications, shows resolution of the central sleep apnea (see figure on p. 168). A 60 second PSG tracing from that study is shown below.

REFERENCES

1. Teichtahl H, Wang D, Cunnington D, *et al*. Ventilatory responses to hypoxia and hypercapnia in stable methadone maintenance treatment patients. *Chest* 2005;**128**:1339–1347.

2. Wang D, Teichtahl H. Opioids, sleep architecture and sleep-disordered breathing. *Sleep Med Rev* 2007;**11**:35–46.

3. Wang D, Teichtahl H, Drummer O, *et al*. Central sleep apnea in stable methadone maintenance treatment patients. *Chest* 2005;**128**: 1348–1356.

4. American Academy of Sleep Medicine. *International Classification of Sleep Disorders, Diagnostic and Coding Manual*, 2nd edn. Westchester, IL: American Academy of Sleep Medicine, 2005.

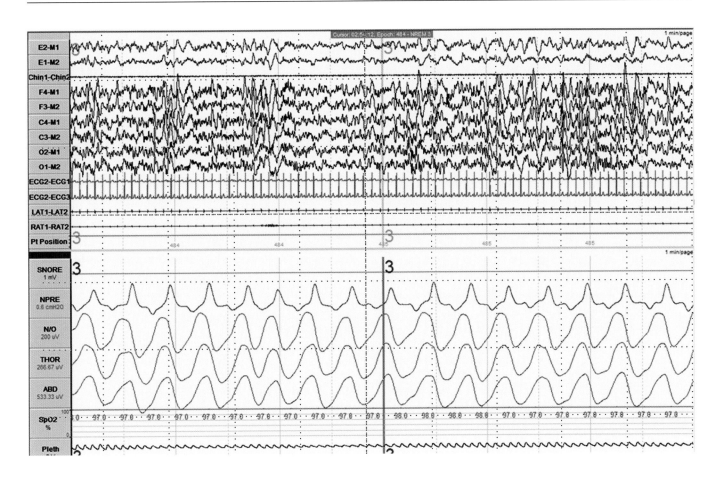

Correct answer: E.

Discussion

A. **Incorrect.** The findings on these epochs fail to show characteristic features of epileptiform activity, such as focal spikes or spike and wave activity.

B. **Incorrect.** While leg EMG activity is increased in this epoch and meets the criteria for a significant leg movement event, this epoch does not display sufficient events to score a series of events characterizing PLMs in sleep.[1]

C. **Incorrect.** The field and polarity of this waveform is atypical for eye movements.

D. **Incorrect.** Hypnagogic hypersynchrony is a pattern of rhythmical and bisynchronous 3–5 Hz waves of high amplitude (75–200 µV). The waves begin abruptly and are widely distributed. They predominate in the anterior, temporal, or posterior leads and may occur intermittently or continuously for several minutes. They are common up to age 2 years, then gradually dissipate; they are rarely seen by age 12 years.

E. **Correct.** These are intermittent trains of high-amplitude bifrontal, synchronous slow waves of 2–3 Hz, often on a background of diffuse slowing of low to medium amplitude. This is a non-specific marker of diffuse encephalopathy, usually metabolic or toxic. Frontal intermittent rhythmic delta activity has also been associated with structural brain lesions affecting midline structures, and increased intraventricular pressure.[2]

REFERENCES

1. Iber C, Ancoli-Israel S, Chesson A for the American Academy of Sleep Medicine. *The AASM Manual for the Scoring of Sleep and Associated Events: Rules, Terminology, and Technical Specifications.* Westchester, IL: American Academy of Sleep Medicine, 2007.

2. Watemberg N, Alehan F, Dabby R, *et al.* Clinical and radiologic correlates of frontal intermittent rhythmic delta activity. *J Clin Neurophysiol* 2002;**19**:535–539.

CASE 52

Correct answer: B.

Discussion

A. **Incorrect**. While the history is positive for seizures, the activity noted on these epochs demonstrate rhythmic increase in EMG tone with minimal change in EEG activity.

B. **Correct**. Vagal nerve stimulation is utilized for refractory epilepsy in adults and children. Respiratory side effects of vagal nerve stimulation include dyspnea, cough, and vocal cord paralysis. Children with snoring and vagal nerve stimulation may warrant evaluation for sleep-disordered breathing based on reports of respiratory pattern changes in sleep.[1] This patient demonstrated no sleep-disordered breathing. However, EEG and EMG activity in a rhythmic pattern was noted, especially in REM sleep.

C. **Incorrect**. Excessive chin and/or limb EMG twitching can be seen on PSG in RBD. Current diagnostic criteria must include either (1) sleep-related injurious, potentially injurious, or disruptive behaviors by history; or (2) abnormal REM sleep behaviors documented during the PSG. The activity seen here is rhythmic, not characteristic of the increased EMG of RBD. Also, the activity is seen in other leads, notably the EEG and ECG (particularly apparent in the 30 second tracing; Fig. 1B), suggestive of artifact rather than EMG activity.

D. **Incorrect**. Individuals taking serotinergic antidepressants can show REM sleep without atonia, identified in submental EMG leads.[2] This pattern would be as noted in C above, not rhythmic as seen here.

E. **Incorrect**. Intermittent artifact would most likely occur at random intervals. The artifact in the EEG, EMG, EOG, and ECG occurs at a regular interval of 25 seconds, as seen in the 90 second epoch (Fig. 1A). The 60 Hz artifact would likely be seen in the effort channels as well.

REFERENCES

1. Nagarajan L, Walsh P, Gregory P, *et al.* Respiratory pattern changes in sleep in children on vagal nerve stimulation for refractory epilepsy. *Can J Neurol Sci* 2003;**30**:224–227.
2. Winkelman J, James L. Serotinergic antidepressants are associated with REM sleep without atonia. *Sleep* 2004;**27**:317–321.

CASE 53

Correct answer: D.

Discussion

A. **Incorrect**. Seizures can occur with sleep initiation, but the activity demonstrated here is insufficient to be characterized as seizure activity as it is without evidence of focal abnormal discharge. Analysis of EEG channels in 10–15 second epochs is often helpful in identification of focal epileptiform activity.

B. **Incorrect**. Hypnagogic jerks, also known as sleep starts, occur on transition from wakefulness to sleep. They are typically sudden, single, brief muscular contractions, and are much briefer in duration than demonstrated on these epochs.

C. **Incorrect**. A sweat artifact is represented by a slow, wandering baseline in the affected lead(s).

D. **Correct**. Body rocking is characteristic of rhythmic movement disorders, which, like hypnagogic jerks, are categorized as sleep–wake transition disorders. The events involve stereotypical body rocking or head banging. They may occur during arousals from sleep and may persist into NREM sleep. They are variable in intensity but can sometimes be violent, causing physical harm.[1]

E. **Incorrect**. Night terrors are periods of partial arousal, typically from slow-wave sleep, unlike that displayed here. They result in high EMG tone and high autonomic activity and are associated with brief periods of confusion and disorientation, occasionally with combativeness and aggressiveness.

REFERENCE

1. Sheldon SH. The parasomnias. In *Principles and Practice of Pediatric Sleep Medicine*, Sheldon SH, Ferber R, Kryger MH (eds.). St. Louis, MO: Elsevier, 2005, pp. 305–315.

CASE 54

Correct answer: E.

Discussion

A. **Incorrect**. RERAs can be scored if there is a fall in signal amplitude with evidence of increased work of breathing.[1] The events demonstrated are, in contrast, associated with lack of respiratory effort.

B. **Incorrect**. Obstructive apneas can be scored only if inspiratory effort is present during the apneic period.[1]

C. **Incorrect**. Cheyne–Stokes breathing is rare in children unless seen in the context of congestive heart failure. For adults, it is scored if there are at least three consecutive cycles of cyclical crescendo–decrescendo change in breathing amplitude and at lease one of the following: (1) five or more central apneas or hypopneas per hour of sleep; or (2) the cyclic crescendo–decrescendo change in breathing amplitude has a duration of at least 10 consecutive minutes.[1] There are no pediatric scoring rules for Cheyne–Stokes breathing. Of note, the events shown are not associated with cyclical crescendo–decrescendo breathing.

D. **Incorrect**. Mixed apneas have absent inspiratory effort in the initial part of the event, but resumption of effort occurs before the end of the event.[1]

E. **Correct**. These central events are defined as a succession of three or more central apneas of > 3 second duration, separated by no more than 20 seconds of normal breathing.[1] Such periodic breathing is common in preterm infants during active/REM and quiet/NREM sleep. Persistence in late infancy and childhood may reflect abnormal brainstem respiratory control, but clear norms are not available.

REFERENCE

1. Iber C, Ancoli-Israel S, Chesson A for the American Academy of Sleep Medicine. *The AASM Manual for the Scoring of Sleep and Associated Events: Rules, Terminology, and Technical Specifications.* Westchester, IL: American Academy of Sleep Medicine, 2007.

CASE 55

Correct answer: A.

Discussion

A. **Correct**. The patient's history of excessive daytime sleepiness dating back to his second decade followed by development of cataplexy, and most recently RBD, is highly suggestive of narcolepsy with cataplexy. The combined hypnogram findings of a SOREM period and frequent nocturnal awakenings and the PSG finding of REM sleep without atonia support this diagnosis.[1,2]

B. **Incorrect**. See C.

C. **Incorrect**. The patient gives a clear history of cataplexy, excluding a diagnosis of idiopathic hypersomnia. Furthermore, the history, PSG, and hypnogram make narcolepsy the more likely diagnosis in this case,[1,3,4] as discussed in A.

D. **Incorrect**. The patient does not give a history of episodic hypersomnia with associated binge eating, hypersexuality, or other behavioral abnormalities with normal functioning in between, excluding a diagnosis of Kleine–Levin syndrome.[3,5]

REFERENCES

1. Billiard M. Diagnosis of narcolepsy and idiopathic hypersomnia. An update based on the International Classification of Sleep Disorders, 2nd edition. *Sleep Med Rev* 2007;**11**:377–388.

2. American Academy of Sleep Medicine. *International Classification of Sleep Disorders, Diagnostic and Coding Manual,* 2nd edn. Westchester, IL: American Academy of Sleep Medicine, 2005.

3. Billiard M, Jaussent I, Dauvilliers Y, Besset A. Recurrent hypersomnia: A review of 339 cases. *Sleep Med Rev* 2011;**15**:247–257.

4. Ali M, Auger RR, Slocumb NL, Morgenthaler TI. Idiopathic hypersomnia: clinical features and response to treatment. *J Clin Sleep Med* 2009;**5**:562–568.

5. AASM. *The International Classification of Sleep Disorders, Diagnostics and Coding Manual.* 2nd edn. Westchester, IL: American Academy of Sleep Medicine, 2005.

Correct answer: D.

Discussion

A. **Incorrect**. While the history is suggestive of this disorder, the actigraphy shown does not demonstrate a stable delay in the major sleep phase, thus excluding this diagnosis.[1]

B. **Incorrect**. The actigraphy does not demonstrate a stable advance in the major sleep phase, which excludes this diagnosis.[1]

C. **Incorrect**. The actigraphy does not demonstrate multiple irregular sleep phases during a 24 hour period, thus excluding this diagnosis.[1]

D. **Correct**. The actigraphy demonstrates sleep and wake times that progressively delay each day, reflecting a period of longer than 24 hours, supporting a diagnosis of free-running or non-entrained circadian rhythm disorder.[1]

REFERENCE

1. American Academy of Sleep Medicine. *International Classification of Sleep Disorders, Diagnostic and Coding Manual*, 2nd edn. Westchester, IL: American Academy of Sleep Medicine, 2005.

Correct answer: A.

Discussion

An MSLT, which should be performed following a standard night-time PSG, is an objective assessment of daytime sleepiness. An MSLT with a short sleep latency and multiple SOREM periods support a diagnosis of narcolepsy with or without cataplexy. Sleep latencies are generally < 5 minutes, but latencies between 6 and 7 minutes have been reported. A small percentage of children with narcolepsy may not have SOREM periods on MSLT. Although not required for a diagnosis of narcolepsy with cataplexy, an MSLT is strongly recommended to confirm the diagnosis and to assess sleepiness objectively. Of note, the MSLT has not been normalized in subjects younger than 8 years of age.

A. **Correct**. Narcolepsy without cataplexy is the most accurate answer. The shown tracing is representative of stage R sleep (REM). The patient, with his clinical history of excessive daytime sleepiness, also meets the objective criteria for narcolepsy, with a sleep latency on MSLT ⩽ 8 minutes and two or more SOREM periods observed following sufficient nocturnal sleep during the night prior. The described episodes of weakness are somewhat suspicious of cataplexy but not "typical." In children, narcolepsy can be considered an evolving disorder in which symptoms, including cataplexy, develop over time. Had the patient described more typical features of cataplexy, the correct diagnosis at this point would be narcolepsy with cataplexy. Since the described episodes are cataplexy-like, the more appropriate diagnosis at this point would be narcolepsy without cataplexy, which may be changed later if the symptoms progress.

B. **Incorrect**. Although excessive daytime sleepiness is a hallmark of idiopathic hypersomnia, both with and without long sleep time, the findings of the MSLT are not consistent with this diagnosis. In idiopathic hypersomnia, an MSLT would be expected to demonstrate a mean sleep latency of < 8 minutes and *fewer* than two SOREM periods, thus differentiating it from narcolepsy findings. Idiopathic hypersomnia is rarely seen prior to adolescence.

C. **Incorrect**. Kleine–Levin syndrome is a rare sleep disorder characterized by recurrent periods of hypersomnia, usually lasting days to weeks, which was not suggested by the history. The syndrome's onset is usually in adolescence and typically is associated with other behavioral abnormalities. It is a clinical diagnosis, not requiring a PSG, which may, in fact, be difficult to perform during symptomatic periods because of behavioral changes. When performed, the results of an MSLT during a symptomatic episode are variable and may include a shortened mean sleep latency and/or two or more SOREM periods.

D. **Incorrect**. Delayed sleep phase disorder is a circadian rhythm sleep disorder in which there is a delay in the phase of the major sleep period in relation to the desired and conventional sleep and wake times. This is not suggested by the patient's history or sleep logs. Further, onset before adolescence is uncommon. The diagnosis is typically made by sleep logs or actigraphy. If performed, MSLT should be analyzed carefully and in the context of patient's misaligned circadian phase. A short mean sleep latency and SOREM periods may be seen, particularly in the earlier nap opportunities if testing is done according to a more conventional schedule.

E. **Incorrect**. Insufficient sleep for a variety of reasons is a common cause of daytime sleepiness in children and adolescents. In this case, sleep logs demonstrated an adequate amount of nocturnal sleep for age and did not demonstrate the "catch-up" sleep one would expect to see on weekends with such a disorder. Although not required for this diagnosis, an MSLT may reveal a short mean sleep latency with or without multiple SOREM periods.

FURTHER READING

American Academy of Sleep Medicine. *International Classification of Sleep Disorders, Diagnostic and Coding Manual*, 2nd edn. Westchester, IL: American Academy of Sleep Medicine, 2005.

Carskadon M, Wolfson A, Acebo C, Tzischinsky O. Adolescent sleep patterns, circadian timing, and sleepiness at a transition to early school days. *Sleep* 1998;**21**:871–881.

Huang Y, Lin Y, Guilleminault C. Polysomnography in Kleine–Levin syndrome. *Neurology* 2008;**70**:795–801.

Kryger M, Roth T, Dement W. *Principles and Practice of Sleep Medicine*, 5th edn. St Louis, MO: Elsevier Saunders, 2011.

Mindell J, Owens J. *A Clinical Guide to Pediatric Sleep: Diagnosis and Management of Sleep Problems*, 2nd edn. London: Lippincott, Williams & Wilkins, 2009.

Question 1

Correct answer: C.

Discussion

A. **Incorrect**. A 60 Hz artifact would demonstrate very fast EEG activity, often obscuring the lead signal.
B. **Incorrect**. This would suggest the presence of ECG electrical activity in a non-ECG lead.
C. **Correct**. As can be seen from both the biocalibration and the stage R sleep images, no identifiable movement is seen in her left eye. This finding was related to her later added history, elicited through questioning by the interpreter of the PSG, of retinoblastoma at a young age with surgical removal of the left eye and replacement with a glass prosthesis.
D. **Incorrect**. This would appear with artifact in all leads referenced to M1.
E. **Incorrect**. This would appear as very slow activity in many or all of the EEG leads.

Question 2

Correct answer: C.

Discussion

A. **Incorrect**. The initial part of the REM is a faster portion, followed by a slower phase.
B. **Incorrect**. Typically the rapid phase of the REM is first, followed by the slow phase.
C. **Correct**. The definition of a REM is that the initial movement of the eye is < 0.5 seconds (whereas the initial phase of a slow eye movement is > 0.5 seconds).
D. **Incorrect**. REMs are typically conjugate in nature.
E. **Incorrect**. REMs can occur in other situations than REM sleep, including reading and scanning the environment when awake.

FURTHER READING

Iber C, Ancoli-Israel S, Chesson A for the American Academy of Sleep Medicine. *The AASM Manual for the Scoring of Sleep and Associated Events: Rules, Terminology, and Technical Specifications*. Westchester, IL: American Academy of Sleep Medicine, 2007.

Correct answer: C.

Discussion

A. **Incorrect**. These findings are compatible with narcolepsy with or without cataplexy, as four SOREM periods occurred. Additional MSLT criteria necessary for this diagnosis would be a mean sleep latency of ≤ 8 minutes on the MSLT.[1]
B. **Incorrect**. Four naps are sufficient to assess for narcolepsy if there are at least two SOREM periods present.[2]

C. **Correct**. As noted above, the four SOREM periods are necessary and specific, although mean sleep latency criteria are also listed as MSLT criteria for this diagnosis in the ICSD.[1]
D. **Incorrect**. The presence of at least 6 hours of sleep on the prior night's PSG and no other sleep disorder noted (e.g. no sleep-disordered breathing) make this a valid PSG to assess for this diagnosis.[1]

REFERENCES
1. American Academy of Sleep Medicine. *International Classification of Sleep Disorders, Diagnostic and Coding Manual*, 2nd edn. Westchester, IL: American Academy of Sleep Medicine, 2005.

2. Littner M, Kushida C, Wise M, *et al.* Practice parameters for clinical use of the Multiple Sleep Latency Test and the Maintenance of Wakefulness Test. *Sleep* 2005;**28**:113–144.

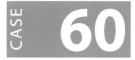

Correct answer: C.

Discussion

These tracings display a pattern of sleep-disordered breathing predominantly in REM sleep (Fig. 1) along with respiratory events in REM sleep (PSG tracing displays hypopneas in REM sleep; Fig. 2).

A. **Incorrect**. With a diagnosis of congestive heart failure, this patient is at risk for Cheyne–Stokes breathing. The mechanism underlying Cheyne–Stokes breathing in part involves suprasensitivity to respiratory disturbance including hyper- and hypocapnia, which results in periodic hypopnea and hyperpnea. During REM sleep, the ventilatory response to both hypoxia and hypercapnia are blunted.[1] Therefore, Cheyne–Stokes breathing is typically less severe or absent in REM sleep compared with NREM sleep.

B. **Incorrect**. Patients with amyotrophic lateral sclerosis do have sleep-disordered breathing, which is often exacerbated during REM sleep.[2] However, in end-stage disease, hypoventilation co-occurs, which would result in REM-related hypercapnia and more consistent rather than periodic REM-related hypopnea. This is inconsistent with the PSG tracing here.

C. **Correct**. REM-related sleep-disordered breathing occurs most commonly in women (a ratio approximately 2:1).

Sleep-disordered breathing is more likely to be confined to REM sleep in younger rather than older women, as older women are more likely to have events in both REM and NREM sleep.[3]

D. **Incorrect**. Children have been shown to have sleep apnea that is generally more severe in REM than in NREM sleep;[4] however, seizures have not been linked to REM-related sleep-disordered breathing, which is the type of sleep-disordered breathing depicted here.

E. **Incorrect**. REM-related sleep-disordered breathing occurs more commonly in women than men.

REFERENCES
1. Douglas NJ, White DP, Weil JV, Pickett CK, Zwillich CW. Hypercapnic ventilatory response in sleeping adults. *Am Rev Resp Dis* 1982;**126**:758–762.
2. Ferguson KA, Strong MJ, Ahmad D, George CF. Sleep-disordered breathing in amyotrophic lateral sclerosis. *Chest* 1996;**110**:664–669.
3. Koo BB, Patel SR, Strohl K, Hoffstein V. Rapid eye movement-related sleep-disordered breathing: influence of age and gender. *Chest* 2008;**134**:1156–1161.
4. Montgomery-Downs HE, O'Brien LM, Gulliver TE, Gozal D. Polysomnographic characteristics in normal preschool and early school-aged children. *Pediatrics* 2006;**117**:741–753.

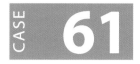

Correct answer: C.

Discussion

A. **Incorrect**. Scoring of hypopnea requires that the breathing decrement be associated with a minimum O_2 desaturation of 3 percentage points, or an arousal, neither of which is present here.

B. **Incorrect**. Central apnea requires a minimum of 10 seconds with absent respiratory effort, which is not the case here.

C. **Correct**. This epoch shows normal breathing during REM sleep. Breathing irregularity and often decrement in airflow and respiratory effort is associated with bursts of REMs in normal phasic REM sleep. In the absence of arousal or desaturation, these breathing decrements are normal.[1]

D. **Incorrect**. Cheyne–Stokes breathing consists of periodic waxing and waning of breathing pattern and is best assessed over epochs of 2 minutes or greater, as at least three consecutive cycles of such breathing are considered diagnostic criteria for this breathing disorder.[2]

REFERENCES

1. Gould GA, Gugger M, Molloy J, *et al*. Breathing pattern and eye movement density during REM sleep in humans. *Am Rev Respir Dis* 1988;**138**:874–877.

2. Iber C, Ancoli-Israel S, Chesson A for the American Academy of Sleep Medicine. *The AASM Manual for the Scoring of Sleep and Associated Events: Rules, Terminology, and Technical Specifications.* Westchester, IL: American Academy of Sleep Medicine, 2007.

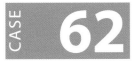

Question 1

Correct answer: C.

Discussion

A. **Incorrect**. While the history is consistent with seizures, this PSG tracing does not demonstrate epileptiform discharges on EEG to suggest the event is a seizure. In order to thoroughly evaluate for seizures, a full 16-channel EEG can be performed as part of the PSG.

B. **Incorrect**. The displayed event occurs out of NREM sleep, not REM sleep. Delta slowing on EEG, indicative of stage N3 sleep, is noted prior to the arousal and event. In RBD, excessive amounts of sustained or intermittent elevation of submental EMG tone or excessive phasic submental or limb EMG twitching during REM sleep would be noted.

C. **Correct**. The event occurs out of stage N3 sleep as delta waves are noted prior to the event, which is characteristic of NREM sleep parasomnias such as sleep-walking. There is a sudden arousal from stage N3 sleep with increased submental EMG tone followed by a mixed alpha and theta EEG activity with resumption of sleep. The fact that the patient does not remember the events and has left the bed to perform a complex motor activity is also consistent with sleep-walking.

D. **Incorrect**. In sleep-related dissociative disorder, EEG wakefulness or alpha rhythm is present before, during, and after the event, which is not the case in this PSG fragment. In the rare instance that a dissociative event occurs after arousal from sleep, there is typically a lag time of at least 15 seconds between EEG arousal and the motor behaviors.

E. **Incorrect**. Nightmares typically occur out of REM sleep, and not NREM sleep as shown in this event. Many times, nightmares are preceded by accelerated heart and respiratory rates or may be associated with increased REMs. In addition, after the nightmare, the patient usually remembers dream content related to the event.

Question 2

Correct answer: B.

Discussion

A. **Incorrect**. Although there is an increase in submental EMG tone, this occurs during NREM sleep, not REM sleep. A K-complex is noted on EEG, signifying stage N2 sleep.

B. **Correct**. The EEG leads referenced to the masseter muscles demonstrate EMG artifact in a phasic pattern at 1 Hz frequency occurring out of stage N2 sleep, as K-complexes are noted in the epoch. According to the AASM Manual, EMG activity must be at least double the existing background activity of the chin EMG channel for a diagnosis of sleep-related bruxism. If the events are phasic in nature, as they are in this case, there must be at least three bursts of increased activity, each 0.25–2 seconds in duration. This is also referred to as rhythmic masticatory muscle activity.[1,2]

C. **Incorrect**. The abnormality in the above fragment is not at 60 Hz frequency.

D. **Incorrect**. The electrode popping artifact is associated with a faulty electrode and should only show in inputs that share the same leads, which is not the case in the epoch shown. The rhythmic activity is noted in all EEG leads referred to both M1 and M2.

E. **Incorrect**. There are no spikes or sharp waves noted on EEG in the PSG fragment to suggest epileptiform activity.

The EEG findings occur at approximately 1 Hz, which is atypical for interictal abnormalities; these usually occur at faster frequencies and are followed by slow waves.

REFERENCES

1. Iber C, Ancoli-Israel S, Chesson A for the American Academy of Sleep Medicine. *The AASM Manual for the Scoring of Sleep and Associated Events: Rules, Terminology, and Technical Specifications.* Westchester, IL: American Academy of Sleep Medicine, 2007.

2. American Academy of Sleep Medicine. *International Classification of Sleep Disorders, Diagnostic and Coding Manual*, 2nd edn. Westchester, IL: American Academy of Sleep Medicine, 2005.

Correct answer: D.

Discussion

A. **Incorrect**. The fragment is showing REM sleep. Sleep-walking typically occurs out of stage N3 sleep, which consists of at least 20% of the epoch showing delta waves on EEG (0.5–2 Hz).[1]

B. **Incorrect**. Although there is increased chin and limb EMG tone noted during REM sleep here, it occurs shortly after a respiratory event. In idiopathic RBD, the increase in chin or limb EMG tone during REM sleep should not be better explained by another sleep disorder (in this case most likely OSA).[2]

C. **Incorrect**. There are no epileptiform discharges noted on this PSG fragment to suggest this diagnosis.

D. **Correct**. OSA can be associated with arousals from REM sleep mimicking symptoms of RBD.[3] This PSG fragment demonstrates an obstructive-appearing respiratory event with O_2 desaturation during REM sleep, followed shortly after by an arousal. Though the patient's overall AHI was only mildly elevated, this was likely a consequence of the decreased amount of total REM sleep time recorded, as the REM sleep AHI was moderately elevated.

E. **Incorrect**. Non-epileptic spells do not typically occur out of sleep but rather occur in wakefulness. They are also not associated with obstructive events during sleep.

REFERENCES

1. Iber C, Ancoli-Israel S, Chesson A for the American Academy of Sleep Medicine. *The AASM Manual for the Scoring of Sleep and Associated Events: Rules, Terminology, and Technical Specifications.* Westchester, IL: American Academy of Sleep Medicine, 2007.

2. American Academy of Sleep Medicine. *International Classification of Sleep Disorders, Diagnostic and Coding Manual,* 2nd edn. Westchester, IL: American Academy of Sleep Medicine, 2005.

3. Iranzo A, Santamaria J. Severe obstructive sleep apnea/hypopnea mimicking REM sleep behavior disorder. *Sleep* 2005;**28**:203–206.

Correct answer: D.

Discussion

A. **Incorrect**. The PSG fragment shows stage N3 sleep and not REM sleep. With RBD, one would expect to see increased chin or limb EMG tone during REM sleep with a history of dream-enactment behavior.

B. **Incorrect**. Panic attacks can occur in NREM sleep but are associated with increased respiratory rate, heart rate, and other associated symptoms, such as palpitations, sweating, shaking, shortness of breath, or dizziness. When occurring out of sleep, the EEG should show an awake (alpha) rhythm and the patient would have recollection of the event.

C. **Incorrect**. Though the history is consistent with seizures, no epileptiform EEG abnormalities are noted on the PSG fragment to suggest this diagnosis. Epileptiform activity, however, cannot be ruled out with the limited montage represented here.

D. **Correct**. Although a typical event was not noted, patients with confusional arousals or NREM sleep parasomnias can have sleep instability with spontaneous arousals following long blocks of stage N3 sleep, as noted in this PSG fragment. Note that the arousal is characteristically preceded and followed by slow-wave (N3) sleep.

E. **Incorrect**. The AHI was reported to be within normal limits, along with normal oxygenation throughout the night. The tracing shows no evidence of sleep-related breathing disorder.

FURTHER READING

American Academy of Sleep Medicine. *International Classification of Sleep Disorders, Diagnostic and Coding Manual,* 2nd edn. Westchester, IL: American Academy of Sleep Medicine, 2005.

Iber C, Ancoli-Israel S, Chesson A for the American Academy of Sleep Medicine. *The AASM Manual for the Scoring of Sleep and Associated Events: Rules, Terminology, and Technical Specifications.* Westchester, IL: American Academy of Sleep Medicine, 2007.

CASE 65

Correct answer: A.

Discussion
A. **Correct.** An electrographic seizure is noted in the left central and left temporal regions (C3 and T3).
B. **Incorrect.** This epoch does not show REM sleep, and RBD is characterized by sustained EMG activity or intermittent loss of REM atonia. Excessive phasic muscle twitching of the submental or limb EMG leads may also be observed.
C. **Incorrect.** The PSG would typically demonstrate recurrent EMG potentials for foot movements, typically at 250–1000 milliseconds duration, with a frequency of 0.3–4.0 Hz in one or both feet; burst potentials longer than the myoclonic range ($\geqslant$ 250 milliseconds) and usually less than 1 second; and trains of at least four bursts.

D. **Incorrect.** The PSG would typically show recurrent and persistent very brief (75 to 150 milliseconds) EMG potentials in various muscles occurring asynchronously and asymmetrically in a sustained manner without clustering. At least 5 potentials every minute should be sustained for at least 20 minutes of stages N2 and N3 sleep.

FURTHER READING
American Academy of Sleep Medicine. *International Classification of Sleep Disorders, Diagnostic and Coding Manual*, 2nd edn. Westchester, IL: American Academy of Sleep Medicine, 2005.
Iber C, Ancoli-Israel S, Chesson A for the American Academy of Sleep Medicine. *The AASM Manual for the Scoring of Sleep and Associated Events: Rules, Terminology, and Technical Specifications*. Westchester, IL: American Academy of Sleep Medicine, 2007.

CASE 66

Correct answer: C.

Discussion

Biot's breathing is a non-periodic breathing pattern characterized by breaths that are irregular in frequency and amplitude, interspersed with central apneas. Biot's breathing is referred to as ataxic breathing by some authors. This pattern was originally described by Biot in a 16-year-old male with tuberculous meningitis.[1] The pathophysiologic mechanisms responsible for this breathing pattern are not clear but are thought to be related to an increased hypoxic drive and decreased hypercapnic ventilatory drive in these individuals.[2] Other types of respiratory disturbance seen in chronic opioid users include cluster breathing, central sleep apnea, OSA, and sleep-related hypoventilation.[3]
A. **Incorrect.** Cheyne–Stokes breathing has a characteristic cyclic crescendo–decrescendo pattern of tidal volume and airflow. The PSG shows at least five central apneas/hypopneas per hour of sleep. Each apnea–hyperpnea cycle usually lasts > 45 seconds. Cheyne–Stokes breathing is characteristically seen in patients with heart failure, stroke, or renal failure.
B. **Incorrect.** Cluster breathing is a periodic breathing pattern, with regular clusters of deep breaths interspersed with central apneas, as illustrated below. The duration of

each cycle is typically shorter than that seen with Cheyne–Stokes breathing, about 30 seconds in this example.
C. **Correct.** The most accurate answer is Biot's breathing (see the discussion). It is the irregular nature of the breathing here that indicates Biot's breathing rather than Cheyne–Stokes breathing or cluster breathing. Biot's breathing may be seen in patients taking chronic opioid medications and, more rarely, in those with medullary brainstem lesions.
D. **Incorrect.** Apneustic breathing, or periodic inspiratory hold, does not fit the pattern shown. This unusual form of disordered breathing has been reported in patients with narcotic abuse, but more commonly in patients with neurologic disorders such as pontine infarct, pontomedullary hemorrhage, multiple sclerosis, Dandy–Walker syndrome, cervical cordotomy, and Rett's syndrome.
E. **Incorrect.** Idiopathic or primary central apnea is not associated with a medical condition or medication such as methadone. Further, the pattern is usually that of an abrupt cessation of breathing with central apneas occurring in a semi-periodic fashion. The duration of each cycle is usually shorter than that seen with Cheyne–Stokes breathing. The breaths do not have a waxing–waning pattern like Cheyne–Stokes breathing or fit the pattern described with cluster breathing above.

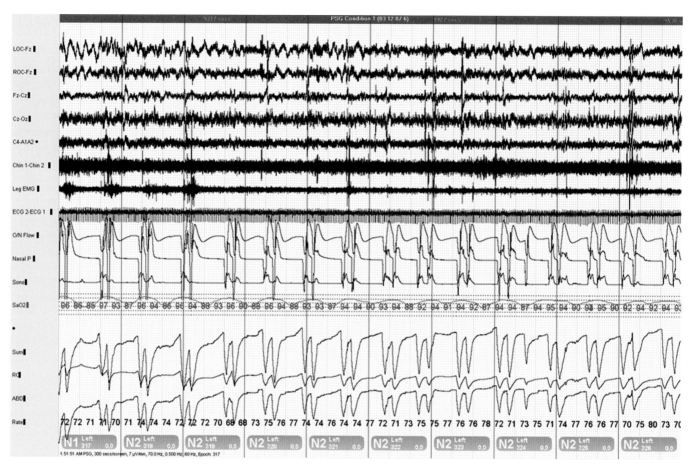

Cluster breathing. Leg EMG, pretibial EMG; LOC-Fpz, left referential EOG; ROC-Fpz, right referential EOG; O/N flow, oronasal airflow; Rate, heart rate; RC, thoracic respiratory effort.

REFERENCES

1. Wijdicks EF. Biot's breathing. *J Neurol Neurosurg Psychiatry* 2007;**78**:512–513.

2. Wang D, Teichtahl H, Drummer O, *et al.* Central sleep apnea in stable methadone maintenance treatment patients. *Chest* 2005;**128**:1348–1356.

3. Farney RJ, Walker JM, Cloward TV, Rhondeau S. Sleep-disordered breathing associated with long-term opioid therapy. *Chest* 2003;**123**: 632–639.

Correct answer: B.

Discussion

A. **Incorrect**. The occurrence of RBD is characterized by dream-enactment, often with loud vocalization and prominent motoric activation, that occurs in REM sleep and is associated with the lack of normal REM atonia. In this case, the behavior did not emerge from REM sleep.

B. **Correct**. Confusional arousal often occurs when a predisposed subject is interrupted by an external stimulus during slow-wave sleep (N3), as was the case here when the technician entered the room to fix the oximeter (see the notes on the figure). Confused behavior associated with some form of vocalization is typical. Episodes may be recurrent or occasional. The O_2 saturation reading proved to be artifactual.

C. **Incorrect.** Sleep terrors and confusional arousal are similar and may occur in the same patient. Both types of parasomnia classically arise from slow-wave sleep, but sleep terror is particularly characterized by intense fear and autonomic activation, with marked difficulty consoling or awakening the patient. In this case, the patient was oriented after only a few minutes of confusion.

D. **Incorrect.** Nocturnal behaviors associated with arousal from slow-wave sleep are often misdiagnosed as panic attacks. Panic attacks can emerge from sleep but predominantly occur during wake and are recurrent in patients with other evidence of an underlying anxiety disorder.

FURTHER READING

American Academy of Sleep Medicine. *International Classification of Sleep Disorders, Diagnostic and Coding Manual*, 2nd edn. Westchester, IL: American Academy of Sleep Medicine, 2005.

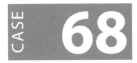

Correct answer: D.

Discussion

A. **Incorrect.** Although the ECG lead is contaminated by movement artifact and the rate recording is not sensing all beats, the ECG remains interpretable and shows important abnormalities, as noted below.

B. **Incorrect.** The arrhythmia following the arousal is not regular nor consistently rapid as would be the case in paroxysmal atrial tachycardia.

C. **Incorrect.** Bradycardia is noted at the end of an obstructive apnea, consistent with a vagal effect during obstruction, but the important abnormality following the arousal is not an artifact.

D. **Correct.** Sinus bradycardia is noted at the end of an obstructive apnea, followed by the sudden onset of atrial fibrillation at the onset of arousal. Sleep apnea is associated with an increased risk of atrial fibrillation and non-sustained ventricular tachycardia. A recent report from the Sleep Health Heart Study reported that the odds of an arrhythmia occurring after a respiratory disturbance were nearly 18 times the odds of an arrhythmia after normal breathing in patients with sleep-disordered breathing.[1]

REFERENCE

1. Monahan K, Storfer-Isser A, Mehra R, *et al.* Triggering of nocturnal arrhythmias by sleep-disordered breathing events. *J Am Coll Cardiol* 2009;**54**:1797–1804.

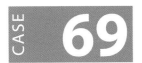

Correct answer: D.

Discussion

A. **Incorrect.** These are moderate frequency, highly regular waveforms that are most likely caused by poor grounding, excessive electrode impedances, dislodged or improper electrode connections, electronic interference (location near electronic devices and power supplies), or long unshielded wires. The artifact in this epoch was > 60 Hz.

B. **Incorrect.** This is a low-frequency artifact that correlates with respiration. It is usually seen in the chin EMG and can be useful to confirm snoring.

C. **Incorrect.** This is a low-amplitude low-frequency waveform that corresponds to the pulse rate. It is caused by the pulsations of the nearby artery, resulting in the electrode movement.

D. **Correct.** The artifact in this epoch is an issue with electrical signaling. The chest belt shows a very fast alternating electrical activity at a rate > 60 Hz. This rate is too high to be physiologic and would, therefore, not be caused by either cardiac or respiratory signals. The artifact is present in the abdominal belt as well as the chest belt but is absent in any of the EEG channels. This suggests that, although the final common pathway for the monitored signals is the head box, the head box itself is not the source of the electrical discharge. When using traditional belts with a strain gauge or Piezo system, displacement of the chest or abdomen is measured but not the change in volume. Accuracy of respiratory assessment is greater when using a respiratory inductance plethysmography system. This system uses a fine wire coil with electrical current, using the impedance of that wire to make realtime assessments of lung volume. In this case, the module used to process the electrical signal was defective and allowed electrical artifact to pass through.

FURTHER READING

Beine B. Troubleshooting and elimination of artifact in polysomnography. *Respir Care Clin North Am* 2005;**11**:617–634.

Chokroverty S, Bhatt M and Goldhammer, T. Polysomnographic recording technique. In *Atlas of Sleep Medicine*, Chokroverty S, Thomas R, Bhatt M (eds.). Philadelphia, PA: Elsevier, 2005, pp. 1–25.

Mazeika GG, Swanson R. *Respiratory Inductance Plethysmography: An Introduction*. Mukilteo, WA: Pro-Tech Services, 2007, pp. 5–9 (http:www.pro-tech.com, accessed 28 February 2012).

CASE 70

Correct answer: B.

Discussion

A. **Incorrect**. A 60 Hz artifact is of moderate frequency, with highly regular waveforms that are most likely caused by poor grounding, excessive electrode impedances, dislodged or improper electrode connections, electronic interference (location near electronic devices and power supplies), and long unshielded wires. Prevention of this artifact can be achieved by the use of shielded wires, proper shielding in the ceilings/walls of patient rooms, keeping impedance low ($< 5 k\Omega$), and ensuring proper electrode connections.

B. **Correct**. Hypnic or hypnagogic foot tremor is a form of rhythmic foot movement that occurs approximately every second for up to several minutes in one or both feet just prior to sleep onset or during light stages of sleep. It may represent a variant of rhythmic movement disorder. It is considered to be a benign disorder with no known sequelae, and there is no known treatment. Note that in this tracing at the beginning of the epoch, nasal airflow is flat and associated with snoring. These findings are consistent with an elevation in upper airway resistance that disrupted

sleep. As the patient transitions back to sleep, the right foot lead shows activity as discussed above.

C. **Incorrect**. The movements seen here occur more frequently than those characteristic of PLMs of sleep. Standard criteria for PLM include their occurrence in a series of four or more movements spaced by intervals of 5 to 90 seconds (onset to onset), with EMG burst durations of 0.5 to 5 seconds.

D. **Incorrect**. Although PSG is not required for the diagnosis of RLS, which is based on the history provided by the patient, prolonged sleep latency as a result of awake PLMs are PSG findings that can be seen in patients with RLS. The frequency of such movements is much less than seen in hypnic foot tremor.

FURTHER READING

Hening WA, Allen RP, Earley CJ, for the Restless Legs Syndrome Task Force of the Standards of Practice Committee of the American Academy of Sleep Medicine. An update on the dopaminergic treatment of restless legs syndrome and periodic limb movement disorder. *Sleep* 2004;**27**:560–583.

Walters AS. Clinical identification of the simple sleep-related movement disorders. *Chest* 2007;**131**:1260–1266.

CASE 71

Correct answer: C.

Discussion

A. **Incorrect**. The patient is not hypoxemic. Further, valsartan and other angiotensin II receptor antagonists are not associated with cough and not known to cause specific PSG abnormalities.

B. **Incorrect**. The patient is not tachycardic, and albuterol is not known to cause specific PSG abnormalities.

C. **Correct**. Citalopram and other SSRIs are associated with a delay in REM onset (as seen here, the REM onset latency is greatly delayed) and a reduction in the duration or even complete absence of REM sleep. These medications are known to increase the number of PLMs, seen in NREM here, and can occur even in patients who have not previously had

complaints of restless legs or limb movements. High REM chin EMG tone and even frank RBD has been associated with SSRI use. Not seen in this recording, frequent NREM-related eye movements have also been reported ("SSRI eyes").

D. **Incorrect**. Lorazepam can cause giant spindles but such spindles are not seen in this recording, and they should be noted in NREM rather than in REM sleep. Alpha intrusion has not been associated with benzodiazepines and these medications are therapy for RLS, not characteristically a cause of PLMs.

FURTHER READING

Roux FJ, Kryger MH. Medication effects on sleep. *Clin Chest Med* 2010;**31**:397–405.

Correct answer: D.

Discussion

A. **Incorrect.** The finding shown by the arrow is cardiac pulsation noted as an artifact in the airflow channel. This is referred to as a cardioballistic artifact in the pressure–flow signal. The respiratory event is central apnea during PAP titration for OSA. The development of central apneas in response to bilevel PAP therapy is often seen in patients with relatively low $Paco_2$ levels and a reduced apneic threshold or CO_2 reserve. The CO_2 reserve is defined as the difference between the resting $Paco_2$ and the value at which there is failure to trigger a breath due to alkalosis. Supplementation with either O_2 or CO_2 has been shown to buffer the CO_2 reserve and reduce central apnea and would be the correct answer regarding resolving the central apnea; however, such treatment would not be expected to directly affect the cardioballistic artifact (see D below).

B. **Incorrect.** As above, this is a cardioballistic artifact caused by cardiogenic oscillations, which are small pulse waves that temporarily correspond to cardiac contractions in the ECG tracing. It is most often observed during exhalation and during central apneic events, as seen in this epoch. There are *no* respiratory efforts during this apnea, nor do cardioballistic waves cause respiratory effort.

C. **Incorrect.** An increase in the IPAP alone is not expected to treat central apneas. A further increase in IPAP may worsen the central apnea, as it did in this patient, as it is likely to cause further hyperventilation and decrease in the $Paco_2$ levels.

D. **Correct.** As above in A, daytime $Paco_2$ is expected to be low, and not elevated, in this patient.

FURTHER READING

Lorenzi-Filho G, Rankin F, Bies I, Douglas Bradley T. Effects of inhaled carbon dioxide and oxygen on Cheyne–Stokes respiration in patients with heart failure. *Am J Respir Crit Care Med* 1999;**159**:1490–1498.

Morrell MJ, Badr MS, Harms CA, Dempsey JA. The assessment of upper airway patency during apnea using cardiogenic oscillations in the airflow signal. *Sleep* 1995;**18**:651–658.

Salloum A, Rowley JA, Mateika JH, *et al.* Increased propensity for central apnea in patients with obstructive sleep apnea: effect of nasal continuous positive airway pressure. *Am J Respir Crit Care Med* 2010;**181**:189–193.

Correct answer: C.

Discussion

A. **Incorrect.** The respiratory events seen in these recordings do not meet the diagnostic criteria for hypopnea, which requires at least a 3 percentage point reduction in O_2 saturation following the respiratory event.[1]

B. **Incorrect.** The respiratory events seen in these epochs are RERAs, which are not associated with an O_2 desaturation that meets criteria for a hypopnea by AASM scoring rules.[1]

C. **Correct.** The presence of an arousal is required for the scoring and diagnosis of RERAs (thus the word "arousal" in the terminology for the event) according to AASM scoring rules.[1] The recommended definition of RERA by the AASM is a sequence of breaths with increasing respiratory effort leading to an arousal from sleep, as shown by progressively more negative esophageal pressure for at least 10 seconds preceding an arousal, with then a resumption of more normal pressures. While these adult rules recommend esophageal manometry to diagnose RERAs, flattening of readings from nasal pressure transducers and/or increasing respiratory effort identified by respiratory inductance plethysmography are also used to detect flow limitation and to diagnose RERAs in clinical practice. These tracings demonstrate such inspiratory flattening, and flutter, of the nasal pressure transducer signal, along with crescendo snoring, preceding an arousal.

D. **Incorrect.** Similar to obstructive apneas and hypopneas, RERAs, as non-apneic or hypopneic upper airway resistance events, can lead to hypersomnia through sleep fragmentation.[2] A RERA index can be calculated to determine the severity of arousals, and the respiratory disturbance index, which includes apneas, hypopneas, and RERAs, determines the frequency of all respiratory events.

REFERENCES

1. Iber C, Ancoli-Israel S, Chesson A for the American Academy of Sleep Medicine. *The AASM Manual for the Scoring of Sleep and Associated Events: Rules, Terminology, and Technical Specifications.* Westchester, IL: American Academy of Sleep Medicine, 2007.

2. Guilleminault C, Stoohs R, Clerk A, *et al.* A cause of excessive daytime sleepiness: the upper airway resistance syndrome. *Chest* 1993; **104**:781–787.

Correct answer: B.

Discussion

A. **Incorrect**. There is no snoring recorded in this epoch (see SNORE channel). These findings are primary events in the legs.

B. **Correct**. PLMs can occur in patients with spinal cord injury.[1] Even in the absence of volitional leg function, it remains important to record limb movements in PSG in such a setting. Numerous treatment options in this setting exist.[2]

C. **Incorrect**. As above, PLMs can occur in patients with spinal cord injury and, therefore, need to be assessed during PSG.

D. **Incorrect**. While the exact mechanisms of PLMs seen in patients with spinal cord injury are not completely understood, both human and animal studies suggest that these movements can be generated in the spinal cord itself, without the involvement of the cortical structures.[3] Spinal cord lesions may lead to limb movements by causing partial disinhibition of the lumbosacral generator, which is enhanced during sleep.[4]

REFERENCES

1. Iber C, Ancoli-Israel S, Chesson A for the American Academy of Sleep Medicine. *The AASM Manual for the Scoring of Sleep and Associated Events: Rules, Terminology, and Technical Specifications*. Westchester, IL: American Academy of Sleep Medicine, 2007, p. 41.

2. de Mello MT, Esteves AM, Tufik S. Comparison between dopaminergic agents and physical exercise as treatment for periodic limb movements in patients with spinal cord injury. *Spinal Cord* 2004;**42**:218–221.

3. Esteves AM, de Mello MT, Lancellotti CL, Natal CL, Tufik S. Occurrence of limb movement during sleep in rats with spinal cord injury. *Brain Res* 2004;**1017**:32–38.

4. Lee MS, Choi YC, Lee SH, Lee SB. Sleep-related periodic leg movements associated with spinal cord lesions. *Mov Disord* 1996;**11**: 719–722.

Correct answer: B.

Discussion

The finding of interest is bruxism.

A. **Incorrect**. This tracing demonstrates bruxism or teeth grinding, seen here in the chin EMG, which is a common parasomnia. The prevalence of bruxism ranges from 20% to 90% in children and declines with age. The prevalence for patients over the age of 60 is less than 5%.

B. **Correct**. While bruxism may occur in any stages of sleep, it is most common in N1 and N2 NREM sleep.

C. **Incorrect**. Patients with bruxism have a normal sleep architecture with normal sleep latency, total sleep time, percentages of sleep stages, and number of arousals. The sleep efficiency is normal, and patients do not usually report poor sleep quality. It should be noted, however, that the tracing here is associated with EEG arousal (note also the increased heart rate at the point of the EEG change).

D. **Incorrect**. The characteristic feature of bruxism is a rhythmic increase (approximately 1 per second) in EMG activity, which is often transmitted to EEG and EOG leads.

FURTHER READING

Lavigne GJ and Manzini C. Bruxism. In *Principles and Practice of Sleep Medicine*, 3rd edn, Kryger M, Roth T, Dement W (eds.). Philadelphia, PA: Saunders, 2000, pp. 773–785.

Lobbezoo F, van der Zaag J, van Selms MK, Hamburger HL, Naeije M. Principles for the management of bruxism. *J Oral Rehabil* 2008; **35**:509–523.

Correct answer: D.

Discussion

A. **Incorrect**. The abnormal finding in the C-FLOW channel represents lack of patient–device synchrony of the inappropriate triggering type (circled in the figure below). The COPD and associated hyperinflation is likely contributing to the inappropriate triggering of the bilevel PAP when the patient has not yet completed the previous breath. Augmenting tidal volume by increasing IPAP might exacerbate this problem by adding to the amount of hyperinflation.

B. **Incorrect**. Augmenting the upper airway patency would be unlikely to reduce the patient–device dyssynchrony as the excess flow is probably generated by lower airway rather than upper airway issues.

C. **Incorrect**. Such an increase would not be transmitted to the patient since the native respiratory rate appears to be faster than 16 breaths/min. Of note, however, maneuvers to increase respiratory rate in this setting would likely result in shorter inhalation times and, because of the expiratory flow limitation in this patient, may result in worsened gas trapping and thus exacerbate the problem.

D. **Correct**. As noted in A (see the circled example in the figure below). By reducing the sensitivity of the flow trigger, extra breaths are less likely to be inappropriately delivered and, therefore, the patient–device dyssynchrony will improve. However, such a maneuver must be done carefully: decreasing the sensitivity has the potential problem of causing the patient, who may have some degree of neuromuscular weakness, to be unable to trigger the bilevel PAP device at all.

FURTHER READING

Tassaux D, Gainnier M, Battisti A, Jolliet P. Impact of expiratory trigger setting on delayed cycling and inspiratory muscle workload. *Am J Respir Crit Care Med* 2005;**172**:1283–1289.

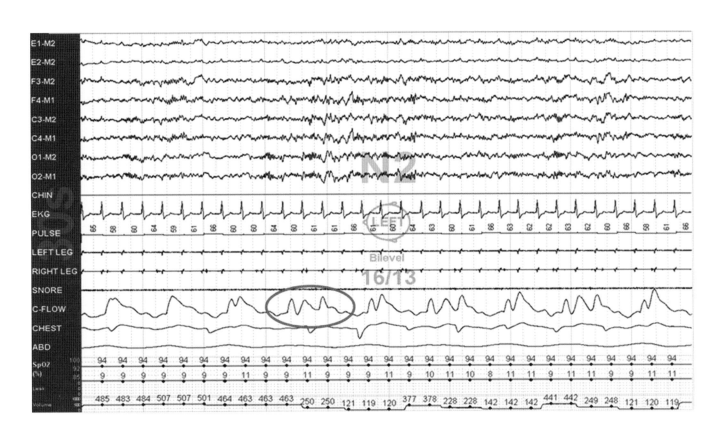

Correct answer: D.

Discussion

A. **Incorrect**. This is not Cheyne–Stokes breathing. There is not a waxing and waning pattern, and the central apneas do not occur in a regular pattern.

B. **Incorrect**. Given her son's diagnosis of a mitochondrial disease, it is most likely that the patient had this mutation as well. Mitochondrial disorders are well known to cause central respiratory events.

C. **Incorrect**. None of the medications listed are known to cause central apnea.

D. **Correct**. Non-invasive ventilation with bilevel PAP in spontaneous/timed mode (i.e. with a back-up rate) has been shown to be an effective therapy in mitochondrial disease with such apnea. The epoch below demonstrates the resolution of sleep-disordered breathing when the patient was placed on bilevel PAP in spontaneous/timed mode with a respiratory rate of 12 breaths/min and bilevel PAP settings of IPAP/EPAP of 15/12 cmH₂O. It is important to note, however, that it still needs to be determined whether non-invasive ventilation alone (as opposed to 24 hour tracheostomy-assisted ventilation) is safe in this setting of severe central apnea.

FURTHER READING

Eckert DJ, Jordan AS, Merchia P, Malhotra A. Central sleep apnea: pathophysiology and treatment. *Chest* 2007;**131**:595–607.

Johnston K, Newth CJ, Sheu KF, *et al*. Central hypoventilation syndrome in pyruvate dehydrogenase complex deficiency. *Pediatrics* 1984;**74**:1034–1040.

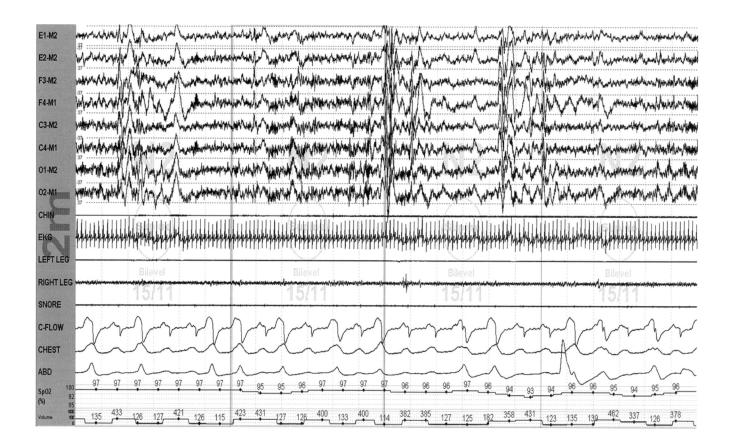

CASE 78

Correct answer: C.

Discussion

A. **Incorrect**. A diagnosis of RLS is made clinically. The patient must meet four clinical criteria: (1) there has to be an urge to move the legs; (2) the urge should happen at night; (3) the urge should happen when at rest; and (4) there has to be a relief in doing so. Approximately 80–90% of patients with RLS have PLMs of sleep. Risk factors for RLS include family history, renal failure, iron deficiency anemia (blood donations, vegetarian diet), neuropathies, and some vitamin deficiencies.

B. **Incorrect**. RBD consists of a combination of the clinical history of violent, potentially or actually injurious behavior during sleep, and concomitant increased muscle tone during REM sleep. This figure does show PLMs of sleep during REM sleep (see EOG), which may occur in severe cases of RLS or PLM disorder, but there was no other history or documented violent behavior at night. Also, the muscle tone in the other chin and right leg leads is normal.

C. **Correct**. PLMs of sleep are the occurrence of limb movements (more commonly legs) during sleep, which fulfill the following criteria: (1) duration between 0.5 and 10 seconds; (2) minimum amplitude of a limb movement is an 8 µV increase in EMG voltage above resting EMG; (3) there has to be at least four limb movements; (4) movements are separated by 5–90 seconds. PLMs of sleep occur in 80–90% of patients with RLS. Approximately 30% of patients in which PLMs of sleep are found have RLS. An index of ⩾ 15/h in adults and ⩾ 5/h in children is closely related to RLS. The term PLM disorder is reserved for those patients with sleep disturbances and significant PLMs of sleep, in which no clinical diagnosis of RLS is made.

D. **Incorrect**. PLMs of wakefulness is the occurrence of limb movements (more commonly legs) during wakefulness. It follows the same criteria as PLMs of sleep. This is REM sleep and not wakefulness.

FURTHER READING

American Academy of Sleep Medicine. *International Classification of Sleep Disorders, Diagnostic and Coding Manual*, 2nd edn. Westchester, IL: American Academy of Sleep Medicine, 2005.

Iber C, Ancoli-Israel S, Chesson A for the American Academy of Sleep Medicine. *The AASM Manual for the Scoring of Sleep and Associated Events: Rules, Terminology, and Technical Specifications*. Westchester, IL: American Academy of Sleep Medicine, 2007.

CASE 79

Correct answer: D.

Discussion

A. **Incorrect**. This 30 second epoch does not represent stage 3 sleep. There are widespread sharply contoured EEG waves overlapping sleep spindles (i.e., stage N2).

B. **Incorrect**. The EEG seems to be normal between the sharply contoured EEG waves observed. The abnormality is also present in many leads and not in only one or two electrodes.

C. **Incorrect**. Bruxism usually carries EMG artifact in the EEG leads. The EMG of bruxism usually shows phasic pattern at 1 Hz frequency lasting 0.25–2 seconds, sustained tonic activity lasting longer than 2 seconds, or a mixed pattern.

D. **Correct**. This EEG tracing shows very frequent epileptiform abnormalities over the right hemisphere that are maximal over the right posterior head regions. There is no involvement of the left hemisphere (Fig. 2 on p. 185). The clinical history is very important to try to differentiate nocturnal seizures from parasomnias. Seizures are usually stereotyped, occurring at any time during the night and sometimes several times a night. Parasomnias are more common in children and usually occur at the same time every night, are not stereotyped, and rarely will occur more than once at night. If suspicion of seizures is high, a full EEG montage must be used.

FURTHER READING

American Academy of Sleep Medicine. *International Classification of Sleep Disorders, Diagnostic and Coding Manual*, 2nd edn. Westchester, IL: American Academy of Sleep Medicine, 2005.

Rodriguez AJ. Pediatric sleep and epilepsy. *Curr Neurol Neurosci Rep* 2007;**7**:342–347.

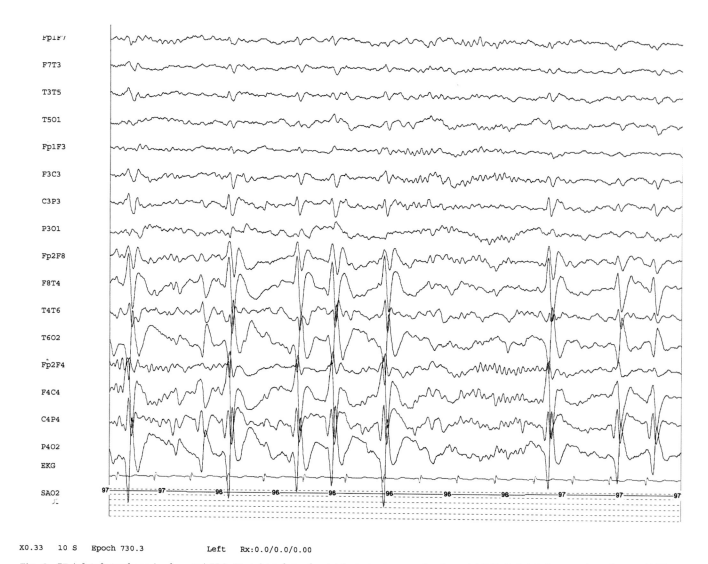

X0.33   10 S   Epoch 730.3   Left   Rx:0.0/0.0/0.00

Fig. 2. F7, left inferior frontal referential EEG; F8, right inferior frontal (anterior temporal) referential EEG; Fp1, left frontopolar referential EEG; Fp2, right frontopolar referential EEG; P3, left parietal referential EEG; P4, right parietal referential EEG; T3, left midtemporal referential EEG; T4, right midtemporal referential EEG; T5, left posterior temporal referential EEG; T6, right posterior temporal referential EEG.

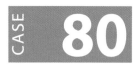

Correct answer: A.

Discussion

A. **Correct.** There is prominent EMG artifact in all EEG leads characteristic of bruxism. The EMG of bruxism usually shows phasic pattern at 1 Hz frequency lasting 0.25–2 seconds, sustained tonic activity lasting longer than 2 seconds, or a mixed pattern. This is a repetitive and sustained activity (mixed pattern), which is severe and associated with a noise of grinding teeth. This is a case of very severe bruxism causing facial pain and at times arousal from sleep, which may lead to fatigue.

B. **Incorrect.** An epileptic seizure involves a synchronic progression of spikes and/or sharp waves with subsequent slowing. There is significant muscle artifact overlapping the EEG shown here, which is otherwise a normal sleep EEG.

C. **Incorrect.** The epoch does not show arousal; however, some bruxism may be accompanied by an arousal.

D. **Incorrect.** Even though bruxism implies muscle artifact in the EEG, it is certainly not just simple muscle artifact in this case.

E. **Incorrect.** The increased muscle artifact occurs out of stage 2 sleep and not REM sleep. Also, the muscle artifact seems to be restricted to the EEG and chin leads.

FURTHER READING

American Academy of Sleep Medicine. *International Classification of Sleep Disorders, Diagnostic and Coding Manual,* 2nd edn. Westchester, IL: American Academy of Sleep Medicine, 2005.

Lavigne G, Rompre P, Montplaisir J. Sleep bruxism: validity of clinical research diagnostic criteria in a controlled polysomnographic study. *J Dent Res* 1996;**75**:546–552.

CASE 81

Correct answer: C.

Discussion

A. **Incorrect.** There is generally low-amplitude EEG signals but there is increased muscle tone in the chin and no REMs. This is NREM stage 1 sleep.

B. **Incorrect.** These limb movements seen in the right leg surface EMG do not meet criteria for PLMs of sleep: the duration is < 0.5 seconds, the separation < 5 seconds, and the amplitude no more than 8 μV above resting EMG.

C. **Correct.** Hypnagogic foot tremor refers to a foot tremor that has a minimum frequency of the EMG burst of 0.3 Hz, a maximal frequency of 4.0 Hz, and a minimum sequence of four bursts. The usual duration of the burst is 250–1000 milliseconds. This phenomenon usually occurs in the transition from wakefulness to sleep or stage 1 or 2 NREM sleep. It has no clinical consequences. This tremor can be observed in only one leg, as seen in the PSG trace.

D. **Incorrect.** Alternating leg muscle activation is another type of leg movement phenomenon. It consists of alternating leg movements (minimum of four) at a frequency of 0.5–3.0 Hz. The usual duration range of the activation is 100–500 milliseconds. No alternating leg movements are seen in this tracing. Alternating leg muscle activation has no known clinical consequences.

E. **Incorrect.** The ECG at times does seem to coincide with the frequency of leg movements, but close inspection reveals that this is not a consistent association in this tracing. Further, the waveform is not typical of ECG artifact as opposed to muscle movement.

FURTHER READING

Berry RB. A woman with rhythmic foot movements. *J Clin Sleep Med* 2007;**3**:749–751.

Iber C, Ancoli-Israel S, Chesson A for the American Academy of Sleep Medicine. *The AASM Manual for the Scoring of Sleep and Associated Events: Rules, Terminology, and Technical Specifications.* Westchester, IL: American Academy of Sleep Medicine, 2007.

CASE 82

Correct answer: B.

Discussion

A. **Incorrect.** The stage is clearly REM sleep. There are REMs with a low-amplitude EEG and generally decreased chin muscle tone. The NREM parasomnias usually occur during the first part of the night and involve more complex behavior, for example sleep-walking, confusional arousal, and night terrors.

B. **Correct.** This epoch shows REM sleep, with bursts of increased muscle tone and twitching (REM without atonia). Children (or adults) can develop RBD as a result of brainstem tumors (or after surgery or radiation), narcolepsy, or use of SSRIs. In adults, the idiopathic form of RBD may progress to an alpha synucleopathy, such as Parkinson's disease, Lewy body dementia, or multiple system atrophy.

C. **Incorrect.** There is no progression of spikes or sharp waves that suggest an epileptic seizure.

D. **Incorrect.** There are muscle twitches and increased muscle tone in REM sleep, but not PLMs that suggest PLMs of sleep.

FURTHER READING

Nevsimalova S, Prihodova I, Kemlink D, Lin L, Mignot E. REM sleep behavior disorder (RBD) can be one of the first symptoms of childhood narcolepsy. *Sleep Med* 2007;**8**:784–786.

Stores G. Rapid eye movement sleep behavior disorder in children and adolescents. *Dev Med Child Neurol* 2008;**50**:728–732.

CASE 83

Correct answer: C.

Discussion

A. **Incorrect.** Bruxism is characterized by muscle artifact involving EEG leads. The EMG of bruxism usually shows a phasic pattern at 1 Hz frequency lasting 0.25–2 seconds, sustained tonic activity lasting longer than 2 seconds, or a mixed pattern.

B. **Incorrect.** At times, this seems like normal stage 2 sleep; however, there is a widespread sharply contoured EEG wave of higher amplitude in both the central and frontal head regions that is projecting to the EOG leads. This activity mimics a K-complex and indeed is very difficult to differentiate without a full EEG montage (see EEG below). Note also that there is an increased beta frequency activity in the EEG, likely related to the stated medication.

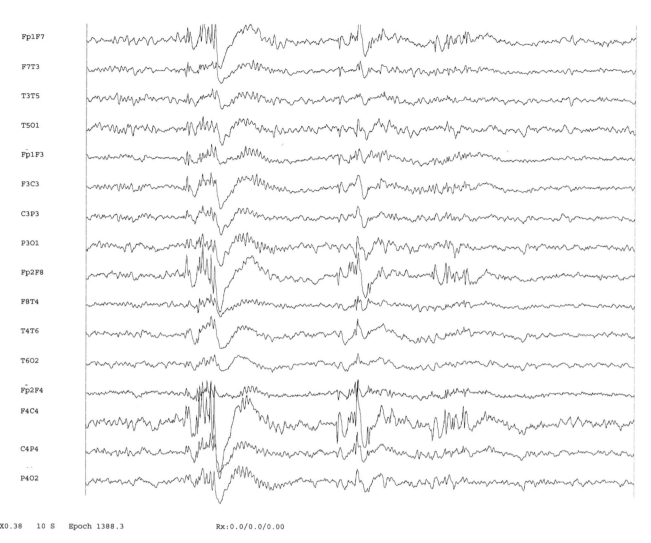

X0.38 10 S Epoch 1388.3   Rx:0.0/0.0/0.00

Fig. 2. F7, left inferior frontal referential EEG; F8, right inferior frontal (anterior temporal) referential EEG; Fp1, left frontopolar referential EEG; Fp2, right frontopolar referential EEG; P3, left parietal referential EEG; P4, right parietal referential EEG; T3, left midtemporal referential EEG; T4, right midtemporal referential EEG; T5, left posterior temporal referential EEG; T6, right posterior temporal referential EEG.

C. **Correct.** If there is clinical suspicion of seizures, a full EEG montage must be used (see below). This widespread sharply contoured EEG activity along with the clinical history makes this suspicious for seizure discharges.

D. **Incorrect.** The EEG between the sharply contoured waves is basically normal. Also, the abnormal waves involve many leads, making this unlikely to be electrode artifact.

Figure 2 shows a full-montage 10 second EEG tracing from the same patient, with generalized spikes and polyspikes and wave discharges of higher amplitude over the frontal head regions. Her dentist placed her on clonazepam under the suspicion of bruxism. Benzodiazepines, such as clonazepam, and phenobarbital have been shown to increase beta frequency activity on the EEG.

CASE **84**

Correct answer: B.

Discussion

A. **Incorrect.** The 30 second PSG epoch shows a markedly increased muscle tone during REM sleep, which along with the clinical history is consistent with idiopathic RBD. Idiopathic RBD is not related to developmental delay but to α-synucleopathy-related degenerative disorders (see B).

B. **Correct**. The clinical and PSG findings are consistent with idiopathic RBD. This disorder is associated with a group of degenerative disorders called synucleopathies, which include Parkinson's disease, Lewy body dementia, and multiple system atrophy. There is accumulation of insoluble α-synuclein protein in some neurons and glial cells. Two thirds of men with this diagnosis over the age of 50 will develop one of these clinical disorders over the course of 13 years.

C. **Incorrect**. Long-acting benzodiazepines, such as clonazepam, are used to treat RBD. However, RBD may be caused by some medications, for example SSRIs.

D. **Incorrect**. There is some muscle artifact in the EEG, which suggests bruxism, but there is increased muscle tone in most of the surface EMG leads. This tracing used extra right and left arm surface EMG leads.

E. **Incorrect**. Brainstem tumors may cause RBD through effects on the pons, where REM sleep originates. However, this patient has no abnormalities on physical examination and has had several years of the disorder. A brain tumor would cause other symptoms of increased intracranial pressure, for example postural headaches (worse lying supine), nausea, vomiting, and focal neurologic signs.

FURTHER READING

American Academy of Sleep Medicine. *International Classification of Sleep Disorders, Diagnostic and Coding Manual*, 2nd edn. Westchester, IL: American Academy of Sleep Medicine, 2005.

Liebman RF, Rodriguez AJ. A patient with epilepsy and new onset of nocturnal symptoms. *Rev Neurol Dis* 2009;**6**:37–38, 40–44.

CASE 85

Correct answer: C.

Discussion

The PSG tracing displays repetitive central apneas in NREM sleep, with mild increases in $ETco_2$ on capnography (the highest CO_2 value on the trace is 46 mmHg) and nadir Spo_2 values of 84%. The PSG, in fact, revealed 228 central apneas, occurring approximately every 20 seconds and seen mostly in NREM sleep. The events were associated with a drop in the respiratory rate to 6 breaths/min and Spo_2 to a nadir of 84%. Neither CO_2 increase to hypoventilation levels nor obstructive events were seen.

A. **Incorrect**. There is no evidence of OSA in this child despite the history of snoring and enlarged tonsils and adenoids.

B. **Incorrect**. While bilevel PAP ventilation may be considered to attempt to immediately control the resultant central sleep apnea and/or desaturation, identification and treatment of the underlying problem is the best definitive strategy. Until then, however, patients with bradypnea and associated hypercapnia may benefit from positive pressure ventilation with a back-up rate (no significant hypoventilation is present here based on the normal CO_2).

C. **Correct**. Because of the high likelihood of an underlying brainstem abnormality given these PSG findings, obtaining an MRI of the brain and brainstem would be the next recommended step for this child.

D. **Incorrect**. While O_2 may be considered as an immediate controlling step, identification and treatment of the underlying problem is the best definitive strategy. Patients with isolated hypoxemia may benefit from supplemental O_2 alone.

E. **Incorrect**.

Follow-up

Indeed, a subsequent MRI revealed a significant Chiari malformation type I. Type I is characterized by herniation of the cerebellar tonsils through the foramen magnum; in Chiari malformation type II, there is also caudal displacement of the vermis, and this is often associated with a myelomeningocele. While often asymptomatic, symptoms of Chiari malformation type I can include headaches, neck pain, ataxia, and sleep-disordered breathing. Findings by PSG can include central and obstructive apnea, bradypnea, and hypoventilation.[1,2]

Treatment of symptomatic Chiari malformation consists of surgical decompression, although this does not always correct the sleep-disordered breathing if the tonsillar herniation has resulted in abnormal development of or injury to the respiratory control neurons in the brainstem.[3]

REFERENCES

1. Dauvilliers Y, Stal V, Abril B, *et al*. Chiari malformation and sleep related breathing disorders. *J Neurol Neurosurg Psychiatry* 2007;**78**:1344–1348.
2. Herschberger ML, Chidekel A. Arnold–Chiari malformation type1 and sleep disordered breathing. *J Pediatr Healthcare* 2003;**17**:190–197.
3. McGirt MJ, Attenello FJ, Atiba A, *et al*. Symptom recurrence after suboccipital decompression for pediatric Chiari: analysis of 256 consecutive cases. *Childs' Nerv Syst* 2008;**24**:1333–1339.

Correct answer: C.

Discussion

A. **Incorrect.** The first actigraph (not shown) indicated a relatively regular bedtime, although wake-up time varied. The second actigraph (Fig. 1) shows generally regular bed and rise time, although the bedtime is later than typical for a 10-year-old child in school. However, the degree of sleepiness and the frequent and late SOREMs would be atypical for this disorder. The history, combined with the regular pattern on actigraphy, is evidence against other circadian rhythm disorders.

B. **Incorrect.** For PLM disorder, the excessive limb movements should not be caused by other concurrent sleep, neurologic, or medical problems; mental disorder; medication; or substance usage. He has PLMs of sleep that are associated with a primary sleep disorder, narcolepsy, possibly exacerbated by low iron stores prior to iron supplementation.

C. **Correct.** The patient's actigraph (Fig. 1) showed consistent onset and offset time for sleep, with adequate sleep of 7–8 hours (except for noted non-use 11/10–11/15/2010). His PSG (Fig. 2) showed improved REM-related sleep-disordered breathing and PLMs and sufficient sleep for MSLT. Results of the MSLT showed mean sleep latency of 1.13 minutes, consistent with pathologic sleepiness (ICSD-2 criteria is a mean sleep latency < 8 minutes for narcolepsy). He also had three out of four naps with SOREM periods (abnormal is two or more). With his chronic daytime sleepiness and PSG findings, he met the diagnostic criteria for narcolepsy. Another alternative to consider would be delayed sleep phase syndrome (note bedtime on actigraphy) with insufficient sleep, leading to reduced sleep latency and also possibly SOREMs on early nap studies. For a 12-year-old child, he gets less than desired total sleep time. However, in his case, the mean sleep latency was severely reduced, and the SOREMs were observed even on the fourth nap study (09:12, 11:05, 13:02, and 15:02). His history of cataplexy was not clear, but children with narcolepsy often will develop cataplexy later in the disease, and the diagnosis should be changed to narcolepsy with cataplexy when that happens. Children with narcolepsy can have significant weight gain at the onset of the disease, which can predispose them to having OSA.[1] Occurrence of RBD is also associated with narcolepsy.[2–4] In addition, PLMs of sleep are associated with both narcolepsy and RBD, which can explain the patient's excessive movement in sleep, as seen in Fig. 1.

D. **Incorrect.** The patient had an abnormal mean sleep latency, and the history for cataplexy was equivocal. Unlike narcolepsy, however, idiopathic hypersomnia is not associated with two or more SOREMs, RBD, or PLMs, as were present in this patient.

E. **Incorrect.** The PSG tracing indeed showed REM sleep without atonia, and review of the PSG with synchronized video showed events of dream-enactment behavior in REM sleep with vocalization. However, since RBD is associated with narcolepsy, the primary diagnosis would be narcolepsy without cataplexy, not RBD as a primary diagnosis.

Additional note

Several other possible diagnoses should be taken into consideration given these findings.

- Behaviorally induced insufficient sleep syndrome. The patient complains of excessive daytime sleepiness, with insufficient sleep time, as indicated in his initial actigraph. However, instead of a delayed sleep phase, he tended to wake up early, with excessive movements in sleep, and did not show any considerably longer sleep time on weekends or holidays, and he continued to complain of sleepiness even when he had sufficient time in bed.
- Restless leg syndrome. In pediatric patients, chronic disturbance of sleep from PLM can predate the diagnosis of definite RLS.[5] Children may not be able to describe the sensory symptoms of RLS. A serum ferritin level should be checked as low iron stores can be associated with RLS and PLM of sleep.
- Kleine–Levin syndrome. He does not have recurrent episodes of hypersomnia. His onset is relatively early for Kleine–Levin syndrome, and he also does not have associated behavioral problems.
- Obstructive sleep apnea. With an overall AHI of 1/h, the patient did not meet the criteria for OSA. However, he did have REM-related sleep-disordered breathing, especially in the supine position, with AHI of 15/h. It should be stressed that children with narcolepsy often can have significant weight gain initially, which predispose them to OSA.
- Sleep-related epilepsy. This could explain the excessive movements in sleep, and the hypersomnolence, but there is no history suggestive of seizure disorder. A 16 channel EEG did not show any epileptiform discharges.

REFERENCES

1. Perriol MP, Cartigny M, Lamblin MD, *et al.* Childhood-onset narcolepsy, obesity and puberty in four consecutive children: a close temporal link. *J Pediatr Endocrinol Metab* 2010;**23**:257–265.

2. Schenck CH, Mahowald MW. Motor dyscontrol in narcolepsy: rapid-eye-movement (REM) sleep without atonia and REM sleep behavior disorder. *Ann Neurol* 1992;**32**:3–10.

3. Nevsimalova S, Prihodova I, Kemlink D, Lin L, Mignot E. REM behavior disorder (RBD) can be one of the first symptoms of childhood narcolepsy. *Sleep Med* 2007;**8**:784–786.

4. Wierzbicka A, Wichniak A, Waliniowska E, *et al.* REM sleep behaviour disorder in narcolepsy. *Neurol Neurochir Pol* 2009;**43**:421–427.

5. Picchietti DL, Stevens HE. Early manifestations of restless legs syndrome in childhood and adolescence. *Sleep Med* 2008;**9**:770–781.

Question 1

Correct answer: B.

Discussion

A. **Incorrect**. Although the airflow (CFLOW) as detected by CPAP device-generated flow signal is reduced to < 10% of baseline for > 10 seconds and, therefore, meets criteria for an apnea, the respiratory event cannot be scored as an obstructive apnea because there is absence of effort during the apnea.[1]

B. **Correct**. The absence of effort during the apnea defines this event as a central apnea.[1]

C. **Incorrect**. A mixed apnea is characterized by absent effort in the initial portion of the apnea that is followed by resumption of inspiratory effort in the latter portion of the apnea, which is not the case here.[1]

D. **Incorrect**. Complex sleep apnea is a condition rather than an event and refers to the phenomenon of emergence of central apneas during CPAP titration of OSA.[2] Although this patient could, therefore, be considered to have complex sleep apnea, the event in question cannot be scored as a complex apnea by current AASM scoring rules.[1]

E. **Incorrect**. The event in question is a true apnea as evidenced by cessation of effort based upon two flow signals, both the abdominal and the chest effort signals.

F. **Incorrect**. Although there is EMG activity in the tibialis EMG signal, there is no evidence of repetitive contractions indicated by phasic EMG activity in the chin EMG channel. Therefore, this is not bruxism. Moreover, bruxism does not typically lead to central apneas, there is no EMG event preceding an arousal, and central apnea as would be expected in a post-arousal (post-sigh) central apnea.

Question 2

Correct answer: E.

Discussion

A. **Incorrect**. The apparent O_2 desaturation from 94 to 80% is not caused by the central apnea in question but by a preceding event that is not visualized in the epochs displayed (and may, in fact, have been a larger degree of desaturation).

B. **Incorrect**. Although O_2 resaturation does appear to occur, this is a consequence of the resumption of breathing – the hyperpnea phase – that is seen at the left corner of the epochs shown, preceding the apneic event in question.

C. **Incorrect**. A desaturation from 97 to 77% does occur following the central apnea in epoch 23, with a significant delay in the nadir of desaturation (approximately 30 seconds). Such a severe, and delayed, O_2 desaturation is rather unusual with central apnea and during CPAP therapy. But this response alone is not the full answer (see E).

D. **Incorrect**. Delayed circulation time is associated with significant delays in O_2 desaturation and appears to be present here. Up to 7 seconds in desaturation delays may be attributable to normal circulation time, and another 7 seconds to delays in signal averaging of a pulse oximeter. However, a delay in desaturation of up to 30 seconds, as in the epochs shown, is correlated with delayed circulation time and cycle length.[3] This response alone is not the correct answer, however, since both C and D are correct.

E. **Correct**. The rationale is outlined in C and D.

F. **Incorrect**. While D is accurate, B is incorrect.

G. **Incorrect**. Both statements are incorrect.

Editor's additional note

While the O_2 desaturation here is often scored, in practice, as the difference between the highest Spo_2 and the nadir Spo_2 surrounding the event, here 97% and 77%, the reader should note that the AASM Manual[1] states that the degree of O_2 desaturation is scored from the "pre-event baseline." Since no such baseline exists here, and in fact the highest Spo_2, 97%, represents the resaturation from the hyperpnea following the response to the preceding event, the apparent O_2 desaturation from 97 to 77% here cannot be assumed to be solely the effect of the central apnea scored, but rather is likely to reflect a combination of events: arousal and hyperpnea from the following event, resumption of sleep and decrease in respiratory drive, and finally the central apnea. Consequently, judging a decrease from 97 to 77% for this central apnea likely overestimates the effect of the central apnea itself.

REFERENCES

1. Iber C, Ancoli-Israel S, Chesson A for the American Academy of Sleep Medicine. *The AASM Manual for the Scoring of Sleep and Associated Events: Rules, Terminology, and Technical Specifications*. Westchester, IL: American Academy of Sleep Medicine, 2007.

2. Gay PC. Complex sleep apnea: it really is a disease. *J Clin Sleep Med* 2008;**4**:403–405.

3. Hall MJ, Xie A, Rutherford R, *et al*. Cycle length of periodic breathing in patients with and without heart failure. *Am J Respir Crit Care Med* 1996;**154**:376–381.

CASE 88

Correct answer: E.

Discussion

A. **Incorrect**. Obstructive apnea requires that the flow (as detected by CPAP device-generated flow signal in this case) be reduced to < 10% of baseline for > 10 seconds and respiratory efforts are seen throughout the apnea event.[1] In this case, there is no effort during the apnea event. Further, the event does not last for 10 seconds. Therefore, this event cannot be scored as an obstructive apnea.

B. **Incorrect**. The absence of effort during an apnea would normally favor a central apnea; however, this patient is not asleep. He is following commands from the technician to hold his breath (see technician's annotation that states, "breath hold" prior to the annotation of "Lights off"). As above, no apnea is present because the event does not last > 10 seconds.

C. **Incorrect**. There is no apnea given the duration of < 10 seconds. Further, a mixed apnea is characterized by absent effort in the initial portion of the apnea that is followed by

resumption of inspiratory effort in the latter portion of the apnea.[1] However, this is not such an event as there is no effort during the entire event.

D. **Incorrect**. There is no evidence that the effort belts are malfunctioning. There are normal excursions and signals prior to and after the "event," without a technician comment or artifacts that denote that the belts were fixed.

E. **Correct**. The patient is following commands from the technician to hold his breath for biocalibration, which is usually performed at the start of the study. Note that in the absence of the technician comment (which states "breath hold"), this event has the appearance of a post-sigh central apnea. Such an event would not have been scored because it occurred during an epoch of wakefulness.

REFERENCE
1. Iber C, Ancoli-Israel S, Chesson A for the American Academy of Sleep Medicine. *The AASM Manual for the Scoring of Sleep and Associated Events: Rules, Terminology, and Technical Specifications*. Westchester, IL: American Academy of Sleep Medicine, 2007.

CASE 89

Correct answer: B.

Discussion

A. **Incorrect**. Although there is a discernible reduction in flow, none of the cardinal features of obstruction are seen. Specifically, there is no evidence for snoring, thoraco-abdominal paradoxic breathing, or inspiratory flow limitation (or flattening) of the inspiratory contour of the CPAP-derived flow signal during the discernible reduction in flow. Admittedly, there is some level of subjectivity in discerning the flattening: one should look for unequivocal signs of inspiratory flow waveform flattening. Interestingly, the flattening can be objectively measured by automated algorithms, which are used in the operation of automatic PAP devices. Moreover, it is important to note that in nasal pressure signals, or device-generated flow signals, appropriate detection of flattening or snoring cannot be achieved without the appropriate sampling frequency, adequately high resolution of the video display, adequate settings of the high and low filters, knowledge about the pressure sensor and any signal preconditioning that it may be conducting, and knowledge of whether the signal is being acquired as a AC or DC channel.

B. **Correct**. Although there is arguably less than 30% reduction in flow, there is greater than 50% reduction in effort belts during the hypopnea events. Such events are not

associated with any of the above-mentioned features of obstruction. The AASM respiratory scoring rules specifically state that a reduction in flow *or* effort that is ≥ 50% compared with baseline and is accompanied by ≥ 3% O_2 desaturation can be scored as an hypopnea as long as it lasts ≥ 10 seconds. It must also be noted, however, that these respiratory scoring rules do not specifically apply to events during the use of PAP. Note also that the crescendo–decrescendo breathing (the decrescendo part being that which is scored as "hypopnea") likely represents the residual periodicity, although without the central apneas, characteristic of patients with heart failure and central sleep apnea.

C. **Incorrect**. The evidence for significant desaturations and reduction in effort belts with periodicity of breathing, and arousals in the EEG associated with these, speak against these tracings being categorized as normal breathing.

D. **Incorrect**. There is no indication that the servo ventilation is malfunctioning based on the epochs depicted, other than to state that crescendo–decrescendo breathing and hypopneas are persisting despite the operation of the servo ventilation. In fact, this is a typical beneficial response, as alluded to above, in that the central apneas are now hypopneas.

E. **Incorrect**. There is no indication that the effort belts are malfunctioning based on the epochs depicted.

CASE 90

Question 1

Correct answer: C.

Discussion

A. **Incorrect**. The respiratory features are not those of stage N1 sleep (see C).
B. **Incorrect**. The respiratory features are not those of stage N2 sleep (see C).
C. **Correct**. The correct response is stage N3. Notice the presence of slow waves in the EEG throughout the epochs diagnostic of N3, and the stable breathing pattern as evidenced by equal tidal volumes, and inspiratory and expiratory times with very little variability. During slow-wave sleep, the respiratory breathing pattern is stabilized with little breathing variability, and is protective against upper airway collapse.
D. **Incorrect**. The respiratory features are not those of stages R sleep (see C).
E. **Incorrect**. The respiratory regularity is uncharacteristic of the awake state.

Question 2

No. The respiratory response is not of help in the scoring as there are no respiratory rules included in the scoring of sleep stages by current AASM rules.[1]

REFERENCE

1. Iber C, Ancoli-Israel S, Chesson A for the American Academy of Sleep Medicine. *The AASM Manual for the Scoring of Sleep and Associated Events: Rules, Terminology, and Technical Specifications.* Westchester, IL: American Academy of Sleep Medicine, 2007.

CASE 91

Correct answer: E.

Discussion

A. **Incorrect**. The patient has indeed developed stage R (REM) sleep as evidenced by the REMs in the beginning of epoch 586. In patients with COPD, REM-sleep-related hypoventilation can occur because the marked hypotonia of intercostal muscles may be contributing to a greater extent to ventilation; these patients experience hyperinflation and reduction in diaphragmatic contribution to ventilation.[1] However, this alone is not the reason for hypoxemia during stage R in patients with COPD and not the only likely cause of the hypoxemia among the choices given.
B. **Incorrect**. Besides the hypoventilation, ventilation–perfusion mismatch also contributes to hypoxemia of REM sleep in patients with COPD.[2] Again, this alone is not the reason for hypoxemia during stage R in patients with COPD and not the only likely cause of the hypoxemia among the choices given.
C. **Incorrect**. As noted in A above, hypoventilation resulting from reduction in accessory muscle contribution to ventilation is an important reason for the hypoxemia that accompanies stage R sleep. There are some breaths that appear to have inspiratory flow limitation in this particular example, and these appear to meet criteria for a hypopnea.[3] Note that hypoventilation is inferred rather than shown here as under current AASM respiratory scoring rules, it cannot be scored without a CO_2 monitor.[3] Hypoventilation alone is not the reason for hypoxemia during stage R in patients with COPD and not the only likely cause of the hypoxemia among the choices given.
D. **Incorrect**. In patients who are receiving non-invasive ventilation, such as the patient described here, mouth opening can occur during stage R sleep through hypotonia of the temporalis muscle; this, in turn, can lead to air leak, ineffective ventilation, and consequent hypoxia. Note the expiratory (negative) portion of the PAP device flow (CFLOW) tracings. There are transient "downward facing" spikes that are indicative of the presence of an air leak.
E. **Correct**. This is the correct response, since all of the above are correct, as noted. The occurrence of stage R sleep, with associated hypotonia and consequent hypoventilation, ventilation–perfusion mismatch, and possible air leak (as evidenced from the spike artifacts in the flow tracing) together most likely contributed to the hypoxemic episode. Again note that hypoventilation can only be inferred here as there is no CO_2 monitor.[3]

REFERENCES

1. White JE, Drinnan MJ, Smithson AJ, Griffiths CJ, Gibson GJ. Respiratory muscle activity during rapid eye movement (REM) sleep in patients with chronic obstructive pulmonary disease. *Thorax* 1995;**50**:376–382.
2. Catterall JR, Calverley PM, MacNee W, *et al.* Mechanism of transient nocturnal hypoxemia in hypoxic chronic bronchitis and emphysema. *J Appl Physiol* 1985;**59**:1698–1703.

3. Iber C, Ancoli-Israel S, Chesson A for the American Academy of Sleep Medicine. *The AASM Manual for the Scoring of Sleep and Associated Events: Rules, Terminology, and Technical Specifications.* Westchester, IL: American Academy of Sleep Medicine, 2007.

CASE 92

Correct answer: C.

Discussion

A. **Incorrect**. The increase in TC_{CO_2} by more than 10 mmHg, compared with the awake baseline value, indicates sleep-related hypoventilation, and in fact the events pictured could be scored as hypoventilation by these criteria.[1] CPAP could induce a rebound of REM sleep, during which central and peripheral chemoreceptor sensitivity is lowest. Without specific assisted ventilation (i.e. bilevel pressure support with inspiratory support above a lower expiratory pressure), hypoventilation could worsen dramatically during REM sleep, leading to worsening hypoxemia.

B. **Incorrect**. Although obstructive events and hypoxemia may improve with CPAP and O_2, this therapy will not address the elevated TC_{CO_2} during sleep and could, in fact, exacerbate the hypoventilation and P_{CO_2}. Assisted ventilation using bilevel PAP is required to address the hypoventilation.

C. **Correct**. The TC_{CO_2} has increased by more than 10 mmHg from awake baseline, indicating that the patient hypoventilates in sleep.[1] In addition to EPAP for OSA (note, however, that the pictured events are not clearly obstructive apneas, as thermistor airflow continues; consequently, if these are hypopneas, they cannot be definitively adjudicated as obstructive), the patient requires adequate pressure support (i.e. IPAP greater than EPAP) to assist with ventilation. Titration goals for EPAP include the elimination of obstructive events, snoring, and airflow limitation. For IPAP, the goals of titration are to prevent further increases in TC_{CO_2} (particularly during REM sleep), improve O_2 saturation, and to attempt to reduce the TC_{CO_2}. To provide adequate ventilatory support, a difference between IPAP and EPAP of 8–10 cmH$_2$O or higher may be required. Note that in some cases supplemental O_2 may need to be added to the bilevel PAP if adequate oxygenation, particularly during REM sleep, is not attained despite otherwise optimal bilevel PAP.

D. **Incorrect**. The goal of servo ventilation is to stabilize oscillatory breathing in patients with Cheyne–Stokes breathing, "complex sleep apnea," and other central apneas. Such ventilation uses the long-term average of the patient's minute ventilation.[2] This patient has hypoventilation. Since ventilatory oscillation is not the pathophysiologic mechanism of sleep-disordered breathing in this patient, the goals of therapy are not specifically met by treatment with servo ventilation. The combination of probable OSA and hypoventilation in this setting suggests the need for bilevel PAP.

E. **Incorrect**. Although the patient is hypoxemic, the awake arterial blood gas reveals little widening of the alveolar–arterial O_2 gradient (and elevated P_{CO_2}), indicating awake alveolar hypoventilation as the cause of the hypoxemia. This is exacerbated during her sleep, although she could also have developed a gas exchange problem during sleep. The addition of O_2 alone could both worsen ventilatory drive and cause decoupling of carboxyhemoglobin molecules (the Haldane effect). Additionally, the patient has untreated OSA and hypoventilation, each of which primarily requires PAP therapy.

Follow-up

The patient was treated with spontaneous-mode bilevel PAP with IPAP/EPAP of 20/10 cmH$_2$O (without supplemental O_2). The following 120 second epoch from REM sleep was recorded later in the split-night study. Note the stabilization of airflow, respiratory effort, and O_2 saturation, and the return of TC_{CO_2} to within 10 torr of baseline.

REFERENCES

1. Iber C, Ancoli-Israel S, Chesson A for the American Academy of Sleep Medicine. *The AASM Manual for the Scoring of Sleep and Associated Events: Rules, Terminology, and Technical Specifications.* Westchester, IL: American Academy of Sleep Medicine, 2007.

2. Teschler H, Dohring J, Wang Y, Berthon-Jones M. Adaptive pressure support servo-ventilation: a novel treatment for Cheyne–Stokes respiration in heart failure. *Am J Respir Crit Care Med* 2001;**164**:614–619.

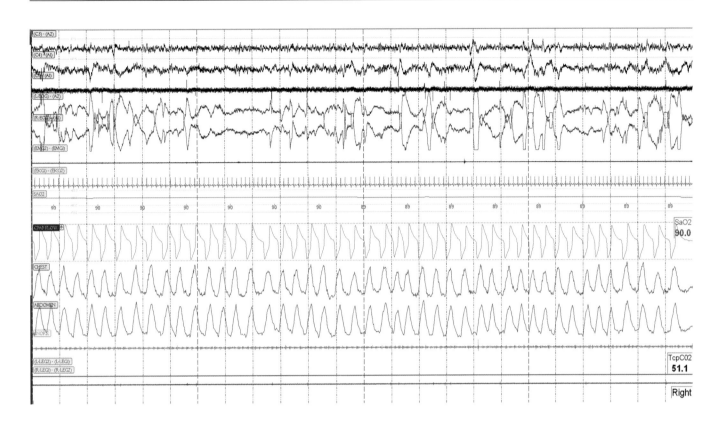

CASE 93

Correct answer: D.

Discussion

A. **Incorrect**. There are no areas of absent or decreased airflow. Oxygen saturation is relatively constant and no discrete O_2 desaturation events are seen.

B. **Incorrect**. The patient is not obese. Although hypoventilation is seen and is most prominent in REM sleep, the patient's abdomen is moving in the opposite direction to both the chest and the flow signals. This paradoxical movement of the diaphragm is most consistent with diaphragmatic weakness.

C. **Incorrect**. The abdomen moves in the opposite direction to the chest, as well as do the thermistor and nasal flow signals. This pattern suggests paradoxical abdominal excursion as a result of diaphragmatic weakness. A spinal cord injury below C5 would not affect diaphragmatic function. An injury at the level of T3 would cause intercostal weakness, which could result in chest movements that were in the opposite direction to the abdomen and flow signals. Thus, the pattern of thoracoabdominal paradox may help to identify the level of a spinal cord lesion.

D. **Correct**. At baseline, the patient has a respiratory acidosis, and the normal alveolar–arterial O_2 gradient suggests that the hypoxemia is a result of hypoventilation while awake. The increase in $TCCO_2$ in sleep indicates that the patient hypoventilates during sleep.[1] No discrete respiratory events are seen, but thoracoabdominal paradox is demonstrated, with paradoxical abdominal movements, and this suggests diaphragmatic weakness.

195

E. **Incorrect**. The patient is hypercapnic while awake, in contrast to patients with Cheyne–Stokes breathing, who are usually hypocapnic as a result of increased chemoresponsiveness.[2] There are no cycles of crescendo–decrescendo changes in breathing amplitude.[1] The sleep-disordered breathing is characterized by a high $TCco_2$ in sleep, with worsening hypoventilation in REM sleep, whereas patients with Cheyne–Stokes respiration typically have lower $TCco_2$ values and worsened sleep-disordered breathing during NREM sleep.[2]

REFERENCES

1. Iber C, Ancoli-Israel S, Chesson A for the American Academy of Sleep Medicine. *The AASM Manual for the Scoring of Sleep and Associated Events: Rules, Terminology, and Technical Specifications.* Westchester, IL: American Academy of Sleep Medicine, 2007.
2. White DP. Pathogenesis of obstructive and central sleep apnea. *Am J Respir Crit Care Med* 2005;**172**:1363–1370.

CASE 94

Correct answer: D.

A. **Incorrect**. Primary or idiopathic central sleep apnea is a rare condition of unknown mechanism, where nocturnal non-invasive ventilation maybe helpful.[1] As this tracing demonstrates central apneas while the patient is on CPAP for OSA, and the patient has symptoms that are characteristic of OSA, this is not the best choice.

B. **Incorrect**. Cheyne–Stokes breathing has a crescendo–decrescendo pattern on respiratory tracings, which is distinguishable from other types of periodic breathing. It is associated primarily with heart failure or neurologic disorders. Assisted nocturnal ventilation with adapt servo devices[2] may improve treatment success.

C. **Incorrect**. Although PLMs are noted on the leg EMG channels, these occur predominantly with arousals in the hyperpneic phase of the periodic breathing. It should be noted that the respiratory events are noted at regular intervals and at times not preceded by arousal, arguing against post-arousal central apneic events, a normal phenomenon.

D. **Correct**. Complex sleep apnea is observed in 6–10% of patients undergoing CPAP titration. In the majority of patients, these improve over time, with persistent events noted in only 2%.[3] These events are secondary to lowering of upper airway resistance and lowering of the $Paco_2$, bringing it closer to the apnea threshold. When this phenomenon is observed, a downward titration or reduction of CPAP pressure is recommended. If these events are persistent during PSG and after use of CPAP, adapt servo ventilation may be considered.[4]

REFERENCES

1. Malhotra A, Owens RL. What is central sleep apnea? *Respir Care* 2010;**55**:1168–1178.
2. Arzt M, Floras JS, Logan AG, for the CANPAP Investigators. Suppression of central sleep apnea by continuous positive airway pressure and transplant-free survival in heart failure: a post hoc analysis of the Canadian Continuous Positive Airway Pressure for Patients with Central Sleep Apnea and Heart Failure Trial (CANPAP). *Circulation* 2007;**115**:3173–3180.
3. Javaheri S, Smith J, Chung E. The prevalence and natural history of complex sleep apnea. *J Clin Sleep Med* 2009;**5**:205–211.
4. Kushida CA, Chediak A, Berry RB, for the Positive Airway Pressure Titration Task Force of the American Academy of Sleep Medicine. Clinical guidelines for the manual titration of positive airway pressure in patients with obstructive sleep apnea. *Clin Sleep Med* 2008;**4**:157–171.

CASE 95

Correct answer: E.

Discussion

A. **Incorrect**. Although propranolol is associated with the development of nightmares,[1] the patient does not have any recollection of her abnormal activity or dream imagery. In addition, the event shown in Fig. 1 is not occurring during REM sleep.

B. **Incorrect**. Paroxetine and other SSRIs have been implicated in drug-induced RBD, which can be reversed by discontinuation of the medication.[2] The patient gives a history of abnormal motor activity. However, the event shown in Fig. 1 is not occurring during REM sleep, and the second PSG epoch (Fig. 2) showing REM sleep does not contain the abnormal elevation of chin EMG tone that is characteristic of RBD.

C. **Incorrect**. Clonazepam is usually the initial treatment for RBD.[3] Although the patient describes abnormal motor activity at night, the patient does not have dream recall, which typically occurs with RBD. Furthermore, Fig. 2 showing REM sleep does not contain the abnormal elevation of chin EMG tone that is characteristic of RBD.

D. **Incorrect**. Pramipexole is indicated for the treatment of RLS.[4] Although there are moderately frequent PLMs of sleep recorded on the PSG, as evidenced by the elevated PLM index, the patient does not give a history consistent with RLS. Nevertheless, it might be inferred that the patient has PLM disorder as a cause of her insomnia complaints. However, PLM disorder is uncommon, and in the presence of sleep-disordered breathing, treatment directed at only PLMs of sleep is generally not necessary.

E. **Correct**. This patient has evidence of moderate sleep-disordered breathing, as demonstrated by her AHI. As shown in Fig. 1, patients with sleep-disordered breathing can terminate episodes of apnea or hypopnea with abnormal motor activity. In the absence of any evidence to suggest an alternative cause of her abnormal motor activity, treatment directed at sleep-disordered breathing

should eliminate these events. An autoPAP study done in the home, in the absence of significant comorbidities, will frequently be able to determine the level of CPAP required to treat this patient's sleep-disordered breathing.[5] Alternatively, a laboratory titration study could be ordered.

REFERENCES

1. McAinsh J, Cruickshank JM. Beta-blockers and central nervous system side effects. *Pharmacol Ther* 1990;**46**:163–197.

2. Parish JM. Violent dreaming and antidepressant drugs: or how paroxetine made me dream that I was fighting Saddam Hussein. *J Clin Sleep Med* 2007;**3**:529–531.

3. Frenette E. REM sleep behavior disorder. *Med Clin North Am* 2010;**94**:593–614.

4. Montagna P, Hornyak M, Ulfberg J, *et al*. Randomized trial of pramipexole for patients with restless legs syndrome (RLS) and RLS-related impairment of mood. *Sleep Med* 2011;**12**:34–40.

5. Morgenthaler TI, Aurora RN, Brown T, for the Standards of Practice Committee of the American Academy of Sleep Medicine. Practice parameters for the use of autotitrating continuous positive airway pressure devices for titrating pressures and treating adult patients with obstructive sleep apnea syndrome: an update for 2007. An American Academy of Sleep Medicine report. *Sleep* 2008;**31**:141–147.

CASE 96

Correct answer: B.

Discussion

A. **Incorrect**. While OSA can be associated with daytime fatigue and unrefreshing sleep, there is no evidence on the two PSG epochs of either apneas or hypopneas. The snore channel does show activity in phase with inspiration, but this finding should be corroborated by documentation of audible snoring by the technician because snoring channels are not usually calibrated.

B. **Correct**. The PSG epochs demonstrate alpha intrusion into NREM sleep. First described by Hauri and Hawkins in 1973,[1] it was linked to fibromyalgia by Moldofsky *et al.* in 1975.[2] Original descriptions were in association with delta (now N3) sleep and it was given the name "alpha-delta sleep." However, alpha intrusion also can be noted in N2 sleep. Apart from in fibromyalgia, alpha intrusion into NREM sleep can be seen in other conditions associated with physical discomfort and, more recently, with the subjective perception of "light" and/or non-restorative sleep and underestimation of total sleep time.[3] It is unclear whether alpha intrusion is an epiphenomenon associated with fibromyalgia and other conditions or that it plays a causal role in disease pathogenesis. Some digital PSG

acquisition systems incorporate spectral analysis software allowing for easy confirmation of the presence of excess alpha activity during NREM sleep.

C. **Incorrect**. Chronic use of benzodiazepines increases both beta and sigma power in the EEG. However, the excess "fast" activity observed on the two PSG epochs provided occurs between 8 and 12 Hz. Both beta and sigma frequencies are faster than 12 Hz.[4]

D. **Incorrect**. While it is possible that chronic fatigue and unrefreshing sleep are symptoms of PLM disorder, the two PSG epochs provided show no evidence of PLMs.

REFERENCES

1. Hauri P, Hawkins DR. Alpha-delta sleep. *Electroenceph Clin Neurophysiol* 1973;**34**:233–237.

2. Moldofsky HD, Scarisbrick P, England R, Smythe H. Musculoskeletal symptoms and non-REM sleep disturbance in patients with "fibrositis syndrome" and healthy subjects. *Psychosom Med* 1975;**37**:341–351.

3. Martinez D, Breitenbach TC, Lenz Mdo C. Light sleep and sleep time misperception: relationship to alpha-delta sleep. *Clin Neurophysiol* 2010;**121**:704–711.

4. Tan X, Uchida S, Matsuura M, Nishihara K, Kojima T. Long-, intermediate- and short-acting benzodiazepine effects on human sleep EEG spectra. *Psychiatry Clin Neurosci* 2003;**57**:97–104.

Correct answer: C.

Discussion

A. **Incorrect**. There is no evidence of seizure activity on the EEG or EMG channels.

B. **Incorrect**. Although there is a decrease in airflow during the vagal nerve stimulator discharge on these tracings, it is not associated with either arousal or O_2 desaturation of at least 3%, at least one of which is required to score a hypopnea.[1]

C. **Correct**. Vagal nerve stimulators are sometimes used to treat medically intractable epilepsy.[2] These are implantable devices that deliver frequent short pulses of electricity to the vagus nerve, which are transmitted upwards into the central nervous system. While the mechanism of action is unclear, it is thought that the electrical impulses modulate central neuronal activity, thereby rendering the patient less susceptible to seizure activity.[3] However, vagal nerve stimulators are also known to bring about a decrease in airflow during their activity, resulting in central apneas and OSA. Hsieh *et al.*[4] published a retrospective review demonstrating the emergence of sleep-disordered breathing in eight out of nine children in whom a vagal nerve stimulator was implanted, including one child who developed an AHI of 37/h, which completely resolved upon inactivation of the vagal nerve stimulator.

D. **Incorrect**, as the child's respiratory effort can clearly be seen to continue throughout the event.

REFERENCES

1. Iber C, Ancoli-Israel S, Chesson A for the American Academy of Sleep Medicine. *The AASM Manual for the Scoring of Sleep and Associated Events: Rules, Terminology, and Technical Specifications.* Westchester, IL: American Academy of Sleep Medicine, 2007.

2. Kabir SM, Rajaraman C, Rittey C, *et al.* Vagus nerve stimulation in children with intractable epilepsy: indications, complications and outcome. *Childs Nerv Syst* 2009;**25**:1097–1100.

3. Hatton KW, McLarney JT, Pittman T, Fahy BG. Vagal nerve stimulation: overview and implications for anesthesiologists. *Anesth Analg* 2006;**103**:1241–1249.

4. Hsieh T, Chen M, McAfee A, Kifle Y. Sleep-related breathing disorder in children with vagal nerve stimulators. *Pediatr Neurol* 2008;**38**:99–103.

Correct answer: D.

Discussion

A. **Incorrect**. The duration of the events is far less than the 0.5–10 second duration required to score PLMs of sleep.[1]

B. **Incorrect**. There is no evidence of any concomitant changes in the respiratory patterns to interpret as a respiratory disturbance here.

C. **Incorrect**. Hypnagogic foot tremor usually occurs during transitions between wake and sleep, or in stages N1 or N2 sleep. The EMG activity seen with hypnagogic foot tremor is usually much longer, 250–1000 milliseconds, and occurs in "trains" of movement lasting 10–15 seconds.[2]

D. **Correct**. According to the 2007 AASM Manual,[1] excessive fragmentary myoclonus is defined by (1) usually a maximum burst duration of 150 microseconds; (2) at least 20 minutes of NREM sleep with these brief twitch-like movements must be recorded; and (3) EMG potentials of at least 5/min must be recorded. Excessive fragmentary myoclonus can be present during wake or sleep, can affect various muscle groups, and often goes unnoticed by the patient. It is appears both in REM and NREM sleep. It is seen mostly in men, and it can be found in 5–10% of patients who present to the sleep laboratory with a complaint of excessive daytime sleepiness. Because excessive fragmentary myoclonus is often seen in the presence of other sleep disorders, its clinical significance remains unclear.[2]

REFERENCES

1. Iber C, Ancoli-Israel S, Chesson A for the American Academy of Sleep Medicine. *The AASM Manual for the Scoring of Sleep and Associated Events: Rules, Terminology, and Technical Specifications.* Westchester, IL: American Academy of Sleep Medicine, 2007.

2. American Academy of Sleep Medicine. *International Classification of Sleep Disorders, Diagnostic and Coding Manual,* 2nd edn: Excessive fragmentary myoclonus. Westchester, IL: American Academy of Sleep Medicine, 2005, pp. 213–215

Correct answer: C.

Discussion

A. **Incorrect**. The tracing shown displays snoring without any respiratory event that fulfills scoring criteria for apnea, hypopnea, RERA, Cheyne–Stokes breathing, or hypoventilation.[1] Use of CPAP is not a first-line therapy for a patient with snoring and no evidence of OSA.[2,3]

B. **Incorrect**. Radiofrequency palate surgery is a modification of uvulopalatopharyngoplasty involving temperature-controlled radiofrequency tissue volume reduction. The long-term effects of radiofrequency palate surgery for the treatment of snoring are uncertain. One study that included 29 patients found a decrease in the median subjective snoring score at 6 months but by 3–4 years only 25% of patients were satisfied with the outcome of the procedure.[4]

C. **Correct**. Weight loss is recommended for obese patients who snore since it may improve snoring and has other health benefits. Sleeping in the lateral position is a low-risk intervention that is warranted in this patient given that his snoring seems to be present when he sleeps in the supine position. This patient should also eliminate alcohol consumption during the several hours prior to sleep.[5]

D. **Incorrect**. The patient gives no indication that he has trouble initiating or maintaining sleep.

Follow-up

Further investigation regarding this patient's complaint of daytime sleepiness is necessary in this situation.

Further note

Mandibular advancement devices may also be considered for the treatment of snoring without evidence of OSA.[6]

REFERENCES

1. Iber C, Ancoli-Israel S, Chesson A for the American Academy of Sleep Medicine. *The AASM Manual for the Scoring of Sleep and Associated Events: Rules, Terminology, and Technical Specifications.* Westchester, IL: American Academy of Sleep Medicine, 2007.

2. Trotter MI, D'souza AR, Morgan DW. Simple snoring: current practice. *J Laryngol Otol* 2003;**117**:164.

3. Kushida CA, Littner MR, Hirshkowitz M, *et al.* Practice parameters for the use of continuous and bilevel positive airway pressure devices to treat adult patients with sleep-related breathing disorders. *Sleep* 2006;**29**:375–380.

4. Hultcrantz E, Harder L, Loord H, *et al.* Long-term effects of radiofrequency ablation of the soft palate on snoring. *Eur Arch Otorhinolaryngol* 2010;**267**:137.

5. Braver HM, Block AJ, Perri MG. Treatment for snoring. Combined weight loss, sleeping on side and nasal spray. *Chest* 1995;**107**:1283.

6. Kushida CA, Morgenthaler TI, Littner MR, *et al.* Practice parameters for the treatment of snoring and obstructive sleep apnea with oral appliances: an update for 2005. *Sleep* 2006;**29**:240–243.

Correct answer: C.

Discussion

The respiratory abnormality is Cheyne–Stokes breathing, with central apneas,[1] and the ICSD-2 classification in this setting is central sleep apnea resulting from Cheyne–Stokes breathing pattern.[2]

A. **Incorrect**. A reanalysis of the data from the largest randomized controlled trial of CPAP in patients with Cheyne–Stokes breathing did show a survival benefit in those participants who had an AHI of < 15/h using CPAP.[3]

B. **Incorrect**. Risk factors include male gender, advanced age, atrial fibrillation and *hypocapnia*.[4]

C. **Correct**. Heart failure accompanied by central sleep apnea with Cheyne–Stokes breathing has been associated with a worse prognosis than heart failure in the absence of, or with a mild form, of such sleep-disordered breathing.[5,6]

D. **Incorrect**. According to the AASM criteria, limb movements should not be scored if they occur during a period from 0.5 seconds preceding an apnea or hypopnea to 0.5 seconds following an apnea or hypopnea.[1]

REFERENCES

1. Iber C, Ancoli-Israel S, Chesson A for the American Academy of Sleep Medicine. *The AASM Manual for the Scoring of Sleep and Associated Events: Rules, Terminology, and Technical Specifications.* Westchester, IL: American Academy of Sleep Medicine, 2007.

2. American Academy of Sleep Medicine. *International Classification of Sleep Disorders, Diagnostic and Coding Manual,* 2nd edn. Westchester, IL: American Academy of Sleep Medicine, 2005.

3. Arzt M, Floras JS, Logan AG, *et al.* Suppression of central sleep apnea by continuous positive airway pressure and transplant-free survival in

heart failure: a post hoc analysis of the Canadian Continuous Positive Airway Pressure for Patients with Central Sleep Apnea and Heart Failure Trial (CANPAP). *Circulation* 2007;**115**:3173–3180.

4. Sin DD, Fitzgerald F, Parker JD, *et al*. Risk factors for central and obstructive sleep apnea in 450 men and women with congestive heart failure. *Am J Respir Crit Care Med* 1999;**160**:1101.

5. Lanfranchi PA, Braghiroli A, Bosimini E, *et al*. Prognostic value of nocturnal Cheyne–Stokes respiration in chronic heart failure. *Circulation* 1999;**99**:1435–1440.

6. Javaheri S, Shukla R, Zeigler H, Wexler L. Central sleep apnea, right ventricular dysfunction, and low diastolic blood pressure are predictors of mortality in systolic heart failure. *J Am Coll Cardiol* 2007;**49**:2028–2034.

CASE 101

Correct answer: D.

Discussion

A. **Incorrect.** While the rhythm during the first portion of the tracing is consistent with normal sinus rhythm, there is a change in the cardiac rhythm upon termination of the obstructive apnea (see D below).

B. **Incorrect.** Normal sinus rhythm is seen in the first portion of the tracing. However, wide complex tachycardia is scored when the rhythm lasts for at least three consecutive beats at a rate greater than 100 bpm, with QRS duration of $\geqslant$ 120 milliseconds.[1] Wide complex QRS morphology is not seen in this tracing.

C. **Incorrect.** In adults, sinus tachycardia is scored for a sustained heart rate of > 90 bpm,[1] which is not observed during the initial portion of the tracing. Atrial fibrillation, which is scored where there is an irregularly irregular ventricular rhythm associated with replacement of consistent P waves by rapid oscillations that vary in size, shape, and timing,[1] is seen at the end of the tracing.

D. **Correct.** Normal sinus rhythm is seen at the beginning of the tracing. Upon termination of the obstructive apnea, the rhythm changes to atrial fibrillation. A retrospective study of over 3000 adults with past or current atrial fibrillation showed that obesity and OSA are independent risk factors for incident atrial fibrillation in individuals younger than 65 years of age.[2]

E. **Incorrect.** As above for C, there is no evidence of tachycardia of any kind during the first portion of the tracing. At the end of the tracing, no P waves are discerned; this is inconsistent with a diagnosis of first-degree AV block, which by definition requires a P wave.

REFERENCES

1. Iber C, Ancoli-Israel S, Chesson A for the American Academy of Sleep Medicine. *The AASM Manual for the Scoring of Sleep and Associated Events: Rules, Terminology, and Technical Specifications*. Westchester, IL: American Academy of Sleep Medicine, 2007.

2. Gami AS, Hodge DO, Herge RM, *et al*. Obstructive sleep apnea, obesity, and the risk of incident atrial fibrillation. *J Am Coll Cardiol* 2007;**49**:565–567.

CASE 102

Correct answer: C.

Discussion

A. **Incorrect.** An ECG artifact can be identified as sharp deflections that consistently coincide with the QRS complex in the ECG lead, not the case here.

B. **Incorrect.** A 60 Hz artifact, caused by environmental electrical interference, is characterized by a uniform sinusoidal waveform at 60 cycles per second, much faster than the frequency observed with electrode popping.

C. **Correct.** This tracing demonstrates repetitive high-voltage deflections in the right EOG and EEG channels. These abrupt deflections usually occur at regular intervals, which often correspond to breathing effort during sleep (as seen for some of the tracing here), secondary to an unstable electrode pulling away from the skin surface. Alternatively, such artifact may also be secondary to excessive drying of the electrode gel. The problematic electrode can be detected by identifying the common electrode in the affected channels, in this case M1 (left mastoid). Recording from an alternative electrode (e.g. M2), adding additional electrode gel, or replacing the affected electrode will likely eliminate this artifact.

D. **Incorrect.** Sweat artifact is characterized by a slow undulating movement of the baseline recording in affected channels caused by perspiration. The frequency and amplitude of this artifact are each usually less than that observed with electrode popping.

CASE 103

Correct answer: D.

Discussion

A. **Incorrect**. An ECG artifact can be identified as sharp deflections that coincide with the QRS complex observed on the ECG lead, and that usually have a much higher frequency (i.e. the heart rate) than that of sweat artifact.

B. **Incorrect**. A 60 Hz artifact is caused by environmental electrical interference and is recognized as a uniform sinusoidal waveform at 60 cycles per second, much faster than the frequency observed with sweat artifact.

C. **Incorrect**. Such artifact is characterized by abrupt high-voltage deflections, typically more abrupt, and of higher voltage than that observed with sweat artifact. Although both electrode popping and sweat artifacts can occur at regular intervals, coinciding with respiration, the frequency of electrode popping is usually faster than that observed with sweat artifact.

D. **Correct**. The EEG and EOG tracings here most clearly show this artifact. The sweat artifact is characterized by a slow undulating movement of the baseline recording in the affected channels. The etiology is perspiration, which alters the potential of the involved electrodes. The slow frequency of sweat artifact may mimic delta waves and lead to over scoring of NREM stage 3 sleep. Uncovering the patient, lowering the room temperature, using a fan on the scalp, or replacing the conductive paste in the electrodes can help to eliminate this artifact.

CASE 104

Correct answer: A.

Discussion

A. **Correct**. The EEG, EOG, and EMG tracings each demonstrate this artifact. This common physiologic artifact is characterized by sharp deflections in the affected channels corresponding to the QRS complex in the ECG lead(s). Such artifact may be avoided by a more cephalad placement of the mastoid electrodes to overlie the mastoid bone instead of the adjacent soft tissue of the neck. Once observed, ECG artifact can also be minimized or eliminated by double referencing the mastoid electrodes. This modification causes cancellation of the ECG voltage vector toward each mastoid electrode. Of additional interest here, the second PSG tracing demonstrates a run of sustained ventricular tachycardia, which persisted for > 30 seconds, thus simultaneously diagnosing ECG artifact and a potentially life-threatening dysrhythmia.

B. **Incorrect**. The 60 Hz artifact is characterized by a uniform sinusoidal waveform at 60 cycles per second, a frequency much faster than that observed with ECG artifact.

C. **Incorrect**. Electrode popping is characterized by repetitive high-voltage deflections, which occur at regular intervals that do not correlate with the ECG lead.

D. **Incorrect**. Sweat artifact is characterized by a slow undulating movement of the baseline recording in affected channels and should not be seen to correlate exactly with the ECG. The frequency of this artifact is markedly slower than that typically observed with ECG artifact.

E. **Incorrect**. Although interictal seizure is suggested by the sharp transients in the EEG derivations, the one-to-one correspondence to the ECG indicates that this is ECG artifact rather than physiologic EEG activity. The non-focal and pervasive nature of the activity, seen in all the EEG, EOG, and even EMG channels, also is highly suggestive of artifact rather than EEG abnormality.

FURTHER READING

Berry RB. *Sleep Medicine Pearls*, 2nd edn. Philadelphia, PA: Hanley& Belfus, 2003, pp. 62–76.

Chokroverty S. *Sleep Disorders Medicine*, 2nd edition. Boston, MA: Butterworth-Heinemann, 1998, pp. 157–181.

Rechtscaffen A, Kales A. *A Manual of Standardized Terminology, Techniques and Scoring System for Sleep Stages of Human Subjects*. Los Angeles, CA: University of California Press, 1968, pp. 1–12.

Verrier RL, Josephson ME. Cardiac arrhythmogenesis during sleep: mechanisms, diagnosis, and therapy. In *Principles and Practice of Sleep Medicine*, Kryger MH, Roth T, Dement WC (eds.). Philadelphia, Elsevier Saunders, 2005, pp. 1171–1179.

Question 1

Correct answer: C.

Discussion

A. **Incorrect**. Amphetamine is not associated with such findings in slow-wave sleep.

B. **Incorrect**. Clomipramine is not associated with such findings in slow-wave sleep.

C. **Correct**. Gamma hydroxybutyrate is approved for use in narcolepsy with cataplexy for the treatment of both excessive daytime sleepiness and cataplexy. It increases sleep consolidation and percentage of slow-wave sleep. Slow-wave sleep is shown in the figure. None associated with this finding.

D. **Incorrect**. Atomoxetine is not associated with such findings in slow-wave sleep.

E. **Incorrect**. Venlafaxine is not associated with such findings in slow-wave sleep.

Question 2

Correct answer: D.

Discussion

A. **Incorrect**. Narcolepsy-cataplexy is associated with RBD but REM sleep is not shown in the figure.

B. **Incorrect**. Sleep terrors, which are accompanied by marked sympathetic activation, are NREM parasomnias arising from slow-wave sleep. She does not display any of the characteristic activities of this disorder here, however.

C. **Incorrect**. Somnambulism (sleep-walking) is also an NREM parasomnia arising from slow-wave sleep. She does not display any of the characteristic activities of sleep-walking.

D. **Correct**. This is a confusional arousal arising during slow-wave (N3) sleep during her CPAP titration. This NREM disorder of arousal usually occurs from slow-wave sleep in the first part of the night. The PSG tracing shows a disturbance from slow-wave sleep. Confusional arousals are marked by mental confusion, disorientation, and confusional behavior. Memory of the event is often impaired. Behavior may become inappropriate. Stress, genetic predisposition, anxiety, insufficient sleep, and psychotropic medication use are among the risk factors/triggers for this disorder, which is most prevalent among children but does occur in an estimated 3–4% of adults.

E. **Incorrect**. Nightmares are manifestations of REM sleep parasomnia, not an NREM parasomnia.

FURTHER READING
Kryger M, Roth T, Dement W. *Principles and Practice of Sleep Medicine*, 5th edn. St Louis, MO: Elsevier Saunders, 2011.

Correct answer: A.

Discussion

A. **Correct**. This is a NREM parasomnia, occurring from slow-wave sleep as shown in this PSG tracing. Sleep terrors typically have a high degree of sympathetic activation, as described here (note the increased heart rate on the ECG at the time of arousal from N3 sleep). Sleep terrors are associated with behavioral manifestations of intense fear; amnesia for the event is common.

B. **Incorrect**. Confusional arousals are also classified as NREM parasomnias but they do not involve the high degree of sympathetic activation that typifies sleep terrors.

C. **Incorrect**. Sleep-walking is also classified as an NREM parasomnia; however, it will typically include ambulation.

D. **Incorrect**. Nightmares are manifestations of REM sleep parasomnia, not NREM parasomnia as displayed here.

E. **Incorrect**. RBD is a REM sleep parasomnia, not an NREM parasomnia as displayed here.

Correct answer: D.

Discussion

A. **Incorrect**. Neurology referral could be considered at a later date if he has recurrent episodes despite treatment of the OSA and his other risk factors for parasomnia. Note that clonazepam may worsen his diathesis for sleep-disordered breathing and should not be used here without definitive OSA treatment.

B. **Incorrect**. There is no indication that he has anger problems in his awake state.

C. **Incorrect**. RBD involves dream enactment, frequently with detailed recall, and typically occurs in the latter portion of the night; it is rare in otherwise healthy young adults.

D. **Correct**. The description of this event fits with an NREM parasomnia such as sleep-walking as it is occurring in the first part of the night and during NREM sleep. The tracing shows representative NREM sleep obstructive apneas with arousals. Triggers for sleep-walking include alcohol consumption, sleep deprivation, stress, and physiologic stress such as full bladder. Risk factors include sleep-disordered breathing. Treatment of the sleep-related breathing disorder is indicated in this setting, as is sleep hygiene and alcohol counseling as these are possible contributors.

E. **Incorrect**. Because injury to self or others is possible with sleep-walking, counseling regarding safety, trigger avoidance, and treatment of risk factors is essential.

Correct answer: E.

Discussion

A. **Incorrect**. The event is better classified as a hypopnea rather than an apnea, as there is continued presence of airflow (seen best in the thermistor) throughout the event. Further, the event does not fit the classic pattern of obstructive apneas seen in OSA, where there would be increasing thoracic and abdominal effort to overcome the upper airway obstruction in addition to increasing diaphragmatic activity during the obstructive event (this is not seen in the tracing). The paradoxic thoracic and abdominal movements here may reflect REM sleep, where the thoracic muscles may be more inhibited than the diaphragm, and/or the neuromuscular weakness of amyotrophic lateral sclerosis, where accessory thoracic muscles may be compensating for the weakened diaphragm. The direction of movement of the chest wall and abdomen in relation to the plethysmography belts is not specified here. However, the paradoxical movement is not specific to the respiratory event shown, as it is present throughout the pictured 2 minutes of REM sleep.

B. **Incorrect**. This is a hypopnea and not an apnea because of the continued presence of airflow throughout the event, as noted in A. Further, this could not be a central apnea as there is persistent thoracic and abdominal effort throughout the event. Additionally, the patient is not stated to be on any medications known to cause respiratory depression.

C. **Incorrect**. The criteria for Cheyne–Stokes breathing are not fulfilled here, since a minimum of three consecutive cycles of cyclical crescendo–decrescendo change in breathing amplitude must be present. Further, Cheyne–Stokes breathing usually has a cycle length of around 60 seconds for a duration of at least 10 minutes, and is less commonly seen during REM sleep periods than in NREM sleep.

D. **Incorrect**. No $Paco_2$ parameter is given during this event to score this as sleep-related hypoventilation (as per the AASM Manual[1]), even though there is evidence of hypoventilation over the course of the night, with the $Paco_2$ rising from 44 mmHg in the evening to 52 mmHg in the morning. Sleep-related hypoventilation typically shows a pattern of prolonged arterial O_2 desaturation, particularly in REM sleep; the current event is more discrete and fulfills parameters for scoring a hypopnea.

E. **Correct**. The tracing in REM sleep shows a hypopnea, with $\geq$ 50% reduction in airflow and associated with a $\geq$ 4% arterial O_2 desaturation. This is associated with minimal diaphragm EMG activity on inspiration, suggesting significant underlying diaphragmatic weakness. There is increased activity on the surface diaphragmatic EMG during expiration, which is likely to represent expiratory muscle activation, with increased activity of the expiratory abdominal muscles at end-expiration. The event is terminated by an arousal, noted by the increased EEG frequency and increase in chin EMG co-incident with the increase in flow. The combination of all the above suggests that this is a hypopnea.

REFERENCE

1. Iber C, Ancoli-Israel S, Chesson A for the American Academy of Sleep Medicine. *The AASM Manual for the Scoring of Sleep and Associated Events: Rules, Terminology, and Technical Specifications.* Westchester, IL: American Academy of Sleep Medicine, 2007.

CASE 109

Question 1

Correct answer: A.

Discussion

A. **Correct**. The respiratory events depicted fit the criteria of the AASM for obstructive apneas and hypopneas. There is a $\geqslant 30\%$ reduction in airflow based on the nasal pressure signal, associated with a $\geqslant 4\%$ arterial O_2 desaturation (recommended apnea and hypopnea rules), with the thoracic band, abdominal band, and diaphragmatic EMG all demonstrating continued effort on at least four occasions over 5 minutes of NREM and REM sleep. The apneas appear obstructive because of continued effort throughout the entire duration of each period of absent airflow, with snoring noises at each hypopnea termination, suggesting (though not diagnosing) an obstructive component for the hypopneas. The frequency of events on this tracing would be sufficient to make a diagnosis of OSA by ICSD-2 criteria if continued at the same rate throughout the total sleep period. The patient is symptomatic from his OSA, as indicated by the Epworth Sleepiness Scale score of 18. Therefore, the diagnosis of OSA is the most consistent at this time and given these data. However, it is important to note that it is unusual to have such significant daytime and nocturnal hypercapnea from severe OSA without significant underlying lung disease or morbid obesity. Note as well that the tracing shown also fits AASM Manual criteria for hypoventilation, which states: "Score hypoventilation during sleep as present if there is a $\geqslant 10$ mmHg increase in $Paco_2$ during sleep in comparison to an awake supine value." The $TCco_2$ monitor displays a $Paco_2$ that reaches 71 mmHg, compared with the awake arterial blood gas derived value for $Paco_2$ of 49 mmHg prior to the study.

B. **Incorrect**. There are no central apneas demonstrated on this tracing. There is continued effort and movement in all events. Further, there is no medication history to support the diagnosis of central sleep apnoea (e.g. narcotics).

C. **Incorrect**. There are no central apneas demonstrated on this tracing. In addition, the events do not have the periodicity and crescendo–decrescendo appearance typical of Cheyne–Stokes breathing.

D. **Incorrect**. There are features, as noted above, that fit criteria for both sleep-related hypoventilation and obstructive apneas (and hypopneas), such that the overall ICSD diagnosis would be most consistent with a diagnosis of OSA (i.e. the disorder here appears better explained by a diagnosis of OSA). One would expect a pattern of prolonged arterial O_2 desaturation in central alveolar hypoventilation, as opposed to the repetitive episodes of desaturation and resaturation that are seen here; these are more fitting with the diagnosis of OSA.

E. **Incorrect**. Although the arterial blood gases and $TCco_2$ levels suggest a diagnosis consistent with a hypoventilation syndrome, the diagnosis of obesity-hypoventilation syndrome cannot be supported in the absence of obesity (normal BMI). The presence of obstructive respiratory events is a frequent finding in the obesity-hypoventilation syndrome.

Question 2

Correct answer: C.

Discussion

A. **Incorrect**. As the hypoventilation persisted despite the likely prevention of upper airway obstruction, this suggests that nocturnal CPAP alone would not be sufficient therapy for this patient.

B. **Incorrect**. Although it is likely that the patient would be able to spontaneously trigger the bilevel device in most NREM sleep stages because of the presence of continuing respiratory effort, the slow spontaneous respiratory rate plus the short central apnoeas in REM sleep make the spontaneous mode less appropriate (see C).

C. **Correct**. The CPAP titration study demonstrated that despite adequate treatment of upper airway obstruction with CPAP there was a significant rise in the $TCco_2$ (100 mmHg) associated with prolonged arterial O_2 desaturation, and hence a diagnosis of sleep hypoventilation would be appropriate based on the tracings shown. The persistence of hypopneas throughout the study at all CPAP pressures tried, in the absence of significant unintentional CPAP leak, is consistent with hypopneas leading to sleep hypoventilation. As the hypoventilation persisted despite the likely prevention of upper airway obstruction, this suggests that nocturnal CPAP alone is insufficient. Interestingly, the summary of the CPAP study night clearly demonstrated a significant rise in $TCco_2$ levels each time the patient entered into sleep, independent of sleep staging, although more marked in slow-wave and REM sleep. The diagnosis of sleep hypoventilation in the absence of upper airway obstruction or a neuromuscular disorder would suggest a problem with control of ventilation causing alveolar hypoventilation during sleep. Furthermore, the evening arterial blood gas showed significant hypercapnea and mild respiratory acidosis, which would suggest that there may be an additional problem with control of ventilation even during wakefulness. The patient appears to require urgent treatment for acute-on-chronic hypercapneic ventilatory failure, particularly in view of the significant end-organ effects noted, such as polycythemia and pulmonary hypertension. Hence, the most appropriate initial management step for this patient would be the institution of bilevel PAP as a high priority. It is likely that the patient would be able to spontaneously trigger the bilevel device in most NREM sleep stages because of the presence of continuing respiratory effort. However, the presence of a slow spontaneous respiratory rate (12–14 breaths/min) with short central apneas in REM sleep shown in the tracing make a spontaneous timed mode of therapy (with an appropriate back-up rate) the most appropriate mode of positive pressure support in the acute setting (answers C correct and B incorrect based on this).

D. **Incorrect.** Given that there are concerns about control of ventilation during wakefulness and sleep, it would be appropriate to perform an MRI of the brain and brainstem to look for a central cause (either cerebral or medullary) for this impairment in the control of ventilation. However, as the patient is in acute-on-chronic hypercapneic ventilatory failure, the most appropriate next management step would be to initiate therapy and *then* to investigate the underlying etiology.

E. **Incorrect.** Given that this patient has an apparent defect in the control of ventilation, it would be appropriate to test his hypercapneic and hypoxic ventilatory responses. If the ventilatory responses are significantly impaired in the absence of any underlying primary neuromuscular disorder (e.g. congenital myopathy, myasthenia gravis), cardiopulmonary disease, or structural brainstem and hindbrain abnormalities, then congenital central hypoventilation syndrome should be considered. This may be confirmed with testing for mutation of *PHOX-2B*, which is linked to occurrence of congenital central hypoventilation syndrome. However, as in answer D, the most appropriate initial step in the acute setting would be to initiate therapy.

Follow-up

Hypercapneic and hypoxic ventilatory responses were subsequently assessed for this patient and showed significant blunting of both responses. Subsequently, a *PHOX2B* analysis was performed, which confirmed that the patient was a heterozygous carrier for the autosomal dominant 20/25 genotype. Consequently, the final diagnosis in this case is most consistent with congenital central hypoventilation syndrome requiring nocturnal ventilatory support, even though an additional diagnosis of OSA has also been made.

CASE 110

Correct answer: E.

Discussion

A. **Incorrect.** The events represent hypopneas with airflow flattening, suggesting residual partial airway obstruction, and this pattern can also be seen during a CPAP titration with inadequate levels of machine pressure. If these events were simply a result of inadequate machine pressure level, however, one would expect a similar appearance, but without the variable leak pattern. In the presence of large leak, as is evident here, the pressure in the pharynx may be much less than that delivered by the machine to the mask. Consequently, the effective pressure delivered to the site of obstruction will be much less than the pressure that would be delivered in a closed system where the unintentional leak was minimized. Therefore, although it is possible that these hypopneas maybe caused by inadequate levels of machine pressure, in this particular case the low pressure at the site of obstruction is likely caused by the large mouth leak (see E) rather than an inadequate pressure delivery to the mask by the CPAP machine. This demonstrates the importance of monitoring CPAP leak when titrating pressure to ensure correct interpretation of the obstructive events. Hence, the most correct answer is that the obstructive hypopnoea is caused by the air leak rather than inadequate machine pressure level. Indeed, in the presence of large air leak, it is not possible to determine the correct machine pressure level.

B. **Incorrect.** The events represent hypopneas, likely obstructive hypopneas, but the pattern of leak seen is more typical of large mouth leak than of large mask leak. Mask leaks tend to be more continuous, with a more constant level of leak, and are not associated with fluctuations in the degree of leak related to arousals. Mask leaks generally do not cause obstructive hypopnoeas, as the pressure in the mask is still effectively delivered to the site of upper airway obstruction.

C. **Incorrect.** The pattern of abnormality seen here does not represent Cheyne–Stokes respiration; it does not have the classic periodicity nor the waxing and waning pattern of Cheyne–Stokes breathing.[1]

D. **Incorrect.** There is no measure of CO_2 and, therefore, no criteria to score hypoventilation, by definition. Although there is persistent desaturation, this is not sufficient to document hypoventilation.[1] Periods of hypoventilation do not normally contain arousals nor demonstrate significant flow limitation (flattening) on the CPAP flow trace. Sleep-related hypoventilation typically shows a pattern of prolonged arterial O_2 desaturation, particularly in REM sleep.

E. **Correct**. The tracing in NREM sleep shows frequent hypopneas on the flow trace, with $\geq 50\%$ reduction in airflow for more than 10 seconds, associated with a $\geq 3\%$ arterial O_2 desaturation and EEG arousal. There are associated reductions in the thoracic and abdominal band excursions consistent with hypopneas. In addition, the CPAP flow trace shows inspiratory flattening of the trace during the hypopneas consistent with flow limitation or obstruction. Each event is terminated by an arousal, noted by the increased EEG frequency and increase in chin EMG co-incident with the increase in flow. The combination of all the above determines that these are hypopneas and, given the flattening of airflow, the hypopneas are likely obstructive events. The CPAP leak trace demonstrates high levels of

unintentional leak (at times $> 30L/min$) during each hypopnea, which falls back to lower levels of leak co-incident with each arousal and increase in CPAP flow. This pattern of intermittent increase in unintentional leak most likely represents intermittent mouth leak in a patient using a nasal-only mask (see discussion to answer B). Therefore, the most correct answer is obstructive hypopneas caused by a mouth leak.

Follow-up

The sleep technologist recognized the mouth leak and entered the patient's room. On further investigation, it was found that the patient had removed a full upper denture prior to going off to sleep. The technologist instructed the patient to replace the upper denture and sleep with it in situ for the rest of the night. A well-fitted chinstrap was also applied. The patient was then allowed to resume sleeping and pressure titration was recommenced. Following application of the chinstrap with the patient's upper denture in place, the problem with mouth leak was largely resolved. At

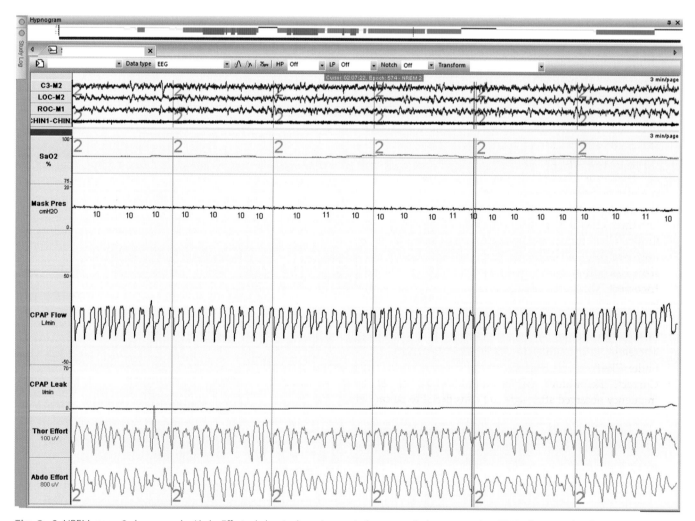

Fig. 2. 2, NREM stage 2 sleep epoch; Abdo Effort, abdominal respiratory inductance plethysmography; CPAP Flow, nasal airflow measured by the CPAP system (L/min); CPAP Leak, derived signal indicating unintentional leak from the CPAP system (L/min); MASK Pres, CPAP pressure (cmH$_2$O) measured at the mask; Thor Effort, thoracic respiratory inductance plethysmography; SaO2 by pulse oximetry.

a pressure of 10 cmH$_2$O, obstructive hypopneas were no longer observed and cortical arousals were reduced. Some flow limitation was still present, but higher pressures were associated with a return of mouth leak. The final conclusion from the study was that CPAP at a pressure of 10 cmH$_2$O largely prevented obstructive events and minimized mouth leak and associated arousals.

A representative 3 minute tracing from NREM sleep where the pressure has been titrated to 10 cmH$_2$O (similar to the

pressure where obstructive hypopneas resulting from the mouth leak were previously observed) is shown in Fig. 2.

REFERENCE

1. Iber C, Ancoli-Israel S, Chesson A for the American Academy of Sleep Medicine. *The AASM Manual for the Scoring of Sleep and Associated Events: Rules, Terminology, and Technical Specifications.* Westchester, IL: American Academy of Sleep Medicine, 2007.

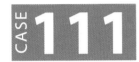

Correct answer: D.

Discussion

A. **Incorrect**. According to the AASM 2007 Manual,[1] Cheyne–Stokes breathing would be scored for at least three consecutives cycles of cyclical crescendo–decrescendo change in breathing amplitude and at least one of the following: (1) five or more central apneas or hypopneas per hour of sleep, and/or (2) the cyclic crescendo–decrescendo change in breathing amplitude has duration of at least 10 consecutive minutes. The shown PSG does not meet these scoring criteria for Cheyne–Stokes breathing. Moreover, Cheyne–Stokes breathing typically occurs in patients with congestive heart failure, and after stroke. In this regard, this subject has no cardiovascular or cerebrovascular history.

B. **Incorrect**. In this sample, as noted above, one can see breathing cessation just after an increased breathing amplitude. While this may be called a post-sigh pause, it has not been defined whether such a post-sigh pause can be scored as central apnea, especially in adults.[1]

C. **Incorrect**. The thermal sensor amplitude does not decrease 90% from baseline in respiratory events after what appear to be a post-sigh pause. In addition, thoracic and abdominal movements are synchronous rather than paradoxic. Therefore, it is unlikely to be residual obstructive apnea under CPAP.

D. **Correct**. Respiratory pauses and/or a slower breath frequency observed after sighs are considered to be caused

by chemomodulation, or Hering–Bruer reflex inhibition of inspiration via vagal stimulation from stretch receptors. Post-sigh breathing behavior may vary depending on genetic background and/or medical condition. Yamauchi et al.[2] have demonstrated that there is a difference in post-sigh breathing pattern between two strains of mice (C57BL/6J and A/J), where the C57BL/6J mice exhibit post-sigh apnea and post-sigh irregular breathing. Moreover, in that study, it was suggested that this strain difference might be explained by the difference in hypercapnic responsiveness (chemosensitivity) and/or overresponse of the Hering–Bruer reflex, which represents high loop gain in these C57BL/6J mice. Consequently, this patient may have hyperchemosensitivity and high loop gain.

E. **Incorrect**. In many patients, a sigh might produce an immediate pause, but it would not influence subsequent breathing.

REFERENCES

1. Iber C, Ancoli-Israel S, Chesson A for the American Academy of Sleep Medicine. *The AASM Manual for the Scoring of Sleep and Associated Events: Rules, Terminology, and Technical Specifications.* Westchester, IL: American Academy of Sleep Medicine, 2007.
2. Yamauchi M, Ocak H, Dostal J, *et al.* Post-sigh breathing behavior and spontaneous pauses in the C57BL/6J (B6) mouse. *Respir Physiol Neurobiol* 2008;**162**:117–125.

Index

TERMS AND CONDITIONS OF USE

1. License

(a) Cambridge University Press grants the customer a non-exclusive license to use this CD-ROM either (i) on a single computer for use by one or more people at different times or (ii) by a single user on one or more computers (provided the CDROM is used only on one computer at one time and is always used by the same user).

(b) The customer must not: (i) copy or authorize the copying of the CD-ROM, except that library customers may make one copy for archiving purposes only, (ii) translate the CD-ROM, (iii) reverseengineer, disassemble, or decompile the CD-ROM, (iv) transfer, sell, assign, or otherwise convey any portion of the CD-ROM from a network or mainframe system.

(c) The customer may use the CD-ROM for educational and research purposes as follows: material contained on a simple screen may be printed out and used within a fair use/fair dealing context; the images may be downloaded for bona fide teaching purposes, but may not be further distributed in any form or made available for sale. An archive copy of the product may be made where libraries have this facility, on condition that the copy is for archiving purposes only and is not used or circulated within or beyond the library where the copy is made.

2. Copyright

All material within the CD-ROM is protected by copyright. All rights are reserved except those expressly licensed.

3. Liability

To the extent permitted by applicable law, Cambridge University Press accepts no liability for consequential loss or damage of any kind resulting from use of the CD-ROM or from errors or faults contained in it.